Ageless Beauty

From The Inside Out

A Simple 10 Step Guide

To Natural Facial Rejuvenation.

by

Kaaren Jordan

www.healingessences.com
(805) 245-9908

© Kaaren Jordan 2011

This book is dedicated to Eileen Poole. Eileen opened me to a new path, based on the work of Dr. Henry Bieler, many years ago, and her continuing guidance supports me still.

I also want to give special thanks for the invaluable support of all my wonderful clients and friends during the creation of this book.

And finally I am especially grateful to my husband, whose hard work, patience, love and faith in me has kept me on track through some very rough roads.

Kaaren Jordan

Table of Contents

Here are the simple steps to help slow the aging process naturally by creating a wellness plan that works for a lifetime:

The 10 Steps

● *Introduction*

Beautiful skin and a youthful appearance start from within. It is simply a reflection of your overall state of health, mirroring the harmony of body, mind and spirit.

This book is offered as a simple guide to help you to create a holistic approach to natural facial rejuvenation and optimal wellness that works over the long haul. These guidelines will give you the tools to look at all aspects of your life as a whole in order to make effective, life long changes.

The process begins by cultivating an understanding of how to balance body, mind and spirit with your individual ever changing needs. The key to maintaining body, mind and spirit harmony is developing self awareness of how your food choices, daily habits and mental-emotional responses to life situations impact your overall well-being. By learning how to choose appropriate foods, balancing your lifestyle, and applying simple self-care tools, you lay the foundation to create vibrant health and ageless beauty for a lifetime. It's never too soon or too late to begin the journey!!

● *Diet . . . You Are What You Eat*

Since our bodies are formed from cells and the quality of the cell is determined by the fuel it receives, diet is where we start.

And so, as many people ask, "What is a healthy diet"?

My reply is that each person as an individual is best served developing an understanding of what are appropriate food choices for their system. This means not only understanding overall balance, but how to re-establish balance when things change under stress, after times of celebration, or after a period of emotional eating. A healthy diet is not a static "one diet fits all" concept, but instead is a more flexible understanding of how to change your choices as your life changes.

Maintaining a health supportive diet requires knowledge of your body's unique needs and how to balance those needs while living life to the fullest. Rigid, unrealistic diets or strict concepts of "good and bad" foods sets us up to fail. They are not helpful in the long run as your needs change according to season, stress levels, travel, social activities, and exercise demands. The foods you chose to eat not only need to fulfill nutritional requirements, but also should consist of readily available choices that fit your lifestyle, and are foods you find satisfying.

The Basics

The following basics are the bare bones on which you can build your own personalized food plan. Everyone is different, and one of the goals of this book is to help you discover what works best for you. The basics are the starting point to build your own optimal diet.

- Increase in your diet lightly cooked (steamed) vegetables

- Eat as much <u>low starch vegetables</u> as you like.

    The following is a partial list:

    Asparagus, Artichoke, Bok Choy, Broccoli, Brussel Sprouts, Cabbage: Napa,Red, Savoy, Cauliflower, Celery, Cilantro , Collards, Cucumber, Dandelion Greens, Endive, Eggplant, Green Beans, Kale, Leeks, Okra, Parsley, Scallions, Snow Peas, Spinach , Squash-Summer, Squash-Yellow, Squash-Zucchini, Swiss Chard, Turnip Greens.

    *Summer Squash and Zucchini are highly recommended. Ample amounts of this group balance your immune system, your PH and assist your "inner healer" to work on regeneration.

1

- Have 2-4 palm size portions of <u>vegetable starch</u> or whole grain a day, depending on your size and activity levels. <u>Do not combine with red meat</u>.

  The following is a partial list:

<u>Vegetable Starch</u>

Carrot, Beets, Corn, Legumes, Potato, Sweet Potato, Yam, Winter Squash: Acorn, Butternut, Hubbard, Spaghetti

<u>Whole Grains</u>

Rice, Spelt, Amaranth, Barley, Buckwheat, Kamut, Millet, Oatbran, Oatmeal, Quinoa, Rye, Wheat

- Include 1-2 palm size portions of <u>protein</u> a day. Choose from the following:

Beef, Lamb, Chicken, Turkey, Fish (no shellfish), Buffalo, Venison (free range, ethically raised, not hormone of additive fed, is best)

- Can have 1-4 free range fertile eggs weekly; treat as <u>protein</u>, <u>do not combine with meat or dairy with the exception of butter</u>.

- Can have 1-2 servings of <u>fruit</u> daily: lightly cooked is better than raw for some people with sensitive digestive systems, when you are stressed, or when you are feeling under par.

- Include 1-2 Tablespoons of oil a day. Choose from the following:

Olive (extra virgin) ,Canola, Grapeseed, Safflower, Sunflower or Apricot Kernel (cold pressed oils are best). Also Hazelnut, Walnut and Flax oils are good but must be fresh and refrigerated, and remember that these oils cannot be heated.

- Eat small regular meals: 3 meals with 1- 2 snacks is a plan most people find works well. The larger meals should be earlier in the day and it is best to avoid overloading at night or eating 2 hours before bed.

• Decrease simple sugars (includes alcohol), simple carbohydrates (flour) and salt; eliminate artificial sweeteners, preservatives and chemicals.

   *Too much of this category dulls and dries the skin from the resulting more acidic PH

• Drink as much pure (non tap) water a day (not with meals) as is comfortable, 6-8 full glasses if possible.

• Eat a wide variety in all the food groups to insure receiving a full spectrum of phyto nutrients

• Bieler's Soup is highly recommended.

   *This soup is referred to as the "Miracle Soup" by many of my clients. They feel and look better with just 1-2 cups a day.

   Ingredients:

   4-6 Zucchini sliced (medium size)

   1 lb Bag Fresh Frozen or Whole Green Beans

   1 Handful of Parsley Tops (No Stems)

   2 Stalks of Celery sliced <u>with strings removed</u> (Optional)

Fill a large pot with 1/3 water and add all the ingredients. Cover and cook in rapidly boiling water for 15-18 minutes until the vegetables are fork tender. Then place all ingredients in blender and puree in batches <u>until smooth</u>. Season with any of your favorite herbs, i.e., paprika, oregano, garlic, lemon or basil. Serve hot or cold. **<u>Do not add salt.</u>**

Food Awareness

It is important to relax for a few minutes both before and after eating. Eating while upset, in a hurry, or while doing something else splits your attention and does not allow you to focus on the experience of enjoying your meals. Eating while stressed, or in a hurry also hinders efficient digestion of your food. Generally it is better to skip a meal rather than 'multi task' while eating

Since digestion begins in the mouth, chew your food thoroughly. Remember to slow down and stop eating before you are completely full. It takes time for the stomach to signal your brain that you've had enough. Quantity changes quality — even too much healthy food can be unhealthy.

It is best to allow at least two hours between your last meal and bedtime, so that your stomach is not full when you go to sleep.

One of the most important points in enjoying food is to release any judgement about foods. Attaching negative thoughts such as guilt over food choices, or adopting a set of rigid rules about eating places unnecessary stress on the entire system by trying to live up to unrealistic goals.

It is important to realize that the idea of "good" and "bad" foods is best viewed as a relative rather than absolute concept. Each of us is biochemically unique with needs that vary in response to our life-style, the seasons, and our environment. So what may be found to be "good" today, may be "bad" next week.

Rather than labeling foods "good" or "bad" on a solely intellectual basis, it may be more productive to release any preconceived judgements and allow your body to guide you towards what is appropriate for you now. A "Body Feedback Journal" is one way to discern what your individual needs are. A sample journal page is given at the end of the diet section.

Food Quality

Always choose foods with the least amount of processing and additives. Avoid all foods that are prepared with chemicals and preservatives, artificial flavorings, colors and sweeteners. Reading labels cannot be overstressed as your best strategy for health supportive eating. Choose Non-GMO foods whenever possible.

Almost every food that is processed has lost vitamins and minerals to some degree and most have salts, fats and sweeteners added to them, further overloading the body.

Buy organic grains, fruits, legumes, and vegetables whenever possible. Raw dairy products, fertile, free-range eggs, and ethically raised, chemical free meats and poultry are your best choices in the animal product category.

Ethically raised, chemical free meats and poultry are in many ways healthier than "factory farmed" animals. Factory farmed animals lead a very stressful existence and accumulate poisons associated with that stress. Because their immune systems are so hampered from stress, they need large amounts of antibiotics and chemicals in their feed which are ultimately passed on to the human consumer. In contrast, ethically raised animals are usually raised in the U.S., and therefore do not contribute to the deforestation of central and South America for grazing land.

Your first and best choice in all food categories is fresh. If for some reason that is not available, frozen organic and standard frozen are the next best option, but always read the labels and check for additives. In a pinch, canned no salt food is better than nothing at all, but again, read the labels carefully. Because our air, soil and ground water is not as pure as it was as little as 30 years ago, it is a prudent idea to eat a wide variety of foods in order to avoid the chemical residues that a specific food would uptake. Even organically grown produce can be affected by the chemicals used previously in the soil, pesticide drift from neighboring farms, and groundwater seepage and rainfall.

Water

Drink as much pure non-tap water as you desire throughout the day. It is best to shoot for at least 6-8 eight ounce glasses daily to hydrate your skin and assist in purifying your entire system. If you are exercising and perspiring or if the weather is warm, increase your intake. Adequate water intake is essential to ensure a healthy body and youthful skin. Large amounts of liquids, of any variety, consumed in conjunction with your meals can hinder digestion and contribute to an uncomfortable bloated feeling, so use moderation here. I find that simply refilling a 32 oz water bottle allows me to keep track of my water intake easily and portably

Eat Seasonally and Locally

Mother nature, in her infinite wisdom, has provided the appropriate foods at the appropriate time of year to keep your body in tune with the seasons and your environment. If the food is in season, grows locally or is from a similar climate zone, it is probably a health-enhancing choice.

Cooking Consciously

The manner in which you prepare your foods and the utensils you cook in all have an affect on the end product. Your preparation time can be used as a break to wind down before eating, so relax and enjoy what you are doing.

To prevent potentially toxic minerals from leaching into your foods, cook in pyrex, corning ware, stainless steel, or lead free earthenware.

Conscious use of cooking techniques can also alter the energetic quality of a food which directly affects the way you feel. Generally speaking, cooking at high temperatures for long periods of time (i.e. baking, roasting, barbecuing) will make foods relatively more energizing and more dry, while stewing over low-heat for a long period of time makes foods more moist and easily digestible. Steaming or parboiling creates a lighter quality and makes foods easier to digest than large amounts of raw foods.

Vegetables

<u>Fresh vegetables should be eaten as the predominant food group in all diets.</u> Vegetables are a store-house of many important vitamins and minerals as well as a great source of fiber. This category can be thought of as the balancers in the nutrition equation.

It is also very important to eat a wide variety of fresh vegetables. Fortunately there are so many varieties   available that one could never become bored. Buy "organically grown" whenever possible or at least wash thoroughly.

The following is partial list:

Green and Low Starch Vegetables

> Alfalfa Sprouts, Other Sprouts, Asparagus, Artichoke, Avocado (in moderation as it is very high in fat), Beet Greens, Bell Peppers, Bok Choy, Broccoli, Brussel Sprouts, Cabbage: Napa, Red, Savoy

> Cauliflower, Celery, Cilantro , Collards, Cucumber, Dandelion Greens, Endive, Eggplant, Garlic , Green Beans,

> Kale Jerusalem Artichokes, Leeks, Mung Bean Sprouts, Mushrooms, Mustard Greens, Radish, Okra, Onions, Parsley, Scallions, Snow Peas

> Spinach , Squash-Summer, Squash-Yellow, Squash-Zucchini, Swiss Chard, Tomato, Turnip Greens, Watercress, Lettuce: Bibb, Butter, Iceberg, Red Leaf, Romaine

Vegetable Starch

> Beet, Legumes, Carrots, Corn, Garbanzo Beans, Jicama, Lentils, Lima Beans, Parsnip, Peas, Potato , Sweet Potato, Turnip, Yam,

> Winter Squash: Acorn, Butternut, Hubbard, Spaghetti

Proteins

The average adult needs far less protein than we are accustomed to consuming. Use all protein sources as side dishes, relying on fresh vegetables and whole grains as the center of your meals. One to two palm sized portions of protein per day (adjusted to individual needs) with at least twice the amount of fresh low starch vegetables and appropriate amounts of grain / starchy vegetables is a health supportive balance. Protein needs vary from person to person, seasonally and according to stress levels, so start low and adjust to what you feel best with.

If you choose to include animal proteins in your diet, buy the leanest cut and remove all visible skin and fat. The fatty portions contain the highest residues of any chemicals, hormones and antibiotics used on the animal as well as being high in saturated fats.

Fish and seafood must be chosen carefully. Be sure to ask where the fish was caught and if they were dipped in antibiotics or preservatives upon catch. When buying canned tuna, be sure to buy "dolphin safe." Because our oceans and lakes are so polluted, only occasional use of bottom feeders, the category of scavenging fish or shellfish is best. Also farm raised fish produces another set of issues because of the manner in which they are raised. Do your research because some farm raised sources are better than others.

The following is a partial list:

> Beef, Beef Liver (organically raised only), Beef Veal, Buffalo, Chicken , Duck, Eggs, Fish, Goose, Lamb, Nuts, Seeds, Tofu, Turkey, Venison.

Grains and Flour Products

Eat a wide variety of grains and make your first choice whole and unprocessed grain. Flour products, even if they are made from whole grains, should be used in moderation. Flour products such as crackers, pastas, and breads usually have salt, fats and many forms of sweeteners added to them, so read labels carefully. Also when grains are milled, vitamins and minerals are lost and natural oils can more easily oxidize. Furthermore, the longer the flour sits before baking, and the longer the finished product sits on the shelf before consumption, the more vitamin loss and oxidation takes place. Grain intake needs to be adjusted to your individual activity level. If you lead a physically active life-style, increase grain portions accordingly.

The following is a partial list:

Grains

> Amaranth, Barley, Buckwheat, Corn, Kamut, Millet, Oatbran, Oatmeal, Quinoa, Rice, Rye, Spelt, Wheat

Breads

Kamut, Spelt, Rye, Millet, Sour Dough, Wheat, Rice Bread, Rice Cakes, Pastas
(yeast free breads are best)

Legumes

Legumes (beans, peas, lentils), properly prepared, are a wonderful non-animal protein source, especially for people with high physical activity levels. If there is a tendency towards digestive problems (i.e. recurrent bloating, indigestion after meals) you may want to use this food group with discretion. It is best to avoid combining legumes with animal protein other than fish or a small amount of dairy.

Legumes can be made more easily digestible if soaked in water overnight and can be cooked in fresh water slowly over low heat for 3-4 hours. Kombu (a type of seaweed popular in Japan) may be added at the beginning of cooking to add flavor and minerals, and make them even more digestible.

As with any protein, be sure to have at least twice the amount of low starch vegetables per serving of protein. Legume amounts may be increased to slightly more than a palm sized portion with an equal amount (or slightly more) of a whole grain and vegetable starch. These proportions again would vary according to individual activity levels.

Fruits

It is always best to eat organic, whole, fresh fruit. Choose what is in season and native to your climate zone. Be sure to wash thoroughly all fruits, especially non-organic. Even though fresh, whole fruit contains a natural form of sugar, this food group should be thought of as a snack or a dessert, not the center of your diet. Dried fruits are a very concentrated form of fruit sugar, so moderation is necessary. Also melons deserve some explanation as they are quite a complex food. If you are experiencing less than optimal health they are best avoided for a time and remember to eat them in season.

The following is a partial list:

Apple, Apricot, Banana, Blackberry, Blueberry, Boysenberry, Cherimoya, Cherry, Cranberry, Dried Fruit, Elderberry , Fig, Gooseberry

Grapefruit, Grapes, Guava, Kiwi, Kumquat, Lemon, Lime, Loganberry, Mango, Nectarine, Orange, Papaya, Peach, Pear

Persimmon, Pineapple, Plum, Pomegranate, Raspberry, Strawberry, Tangerine

Dairy Products*

When using dairy products your first choice should be raw, low-fat in some cases, and low sodium as applicable. Include a variety of plain cultured dairy products like yogurt and kefir to balance intestinal flora. Healthy elimination enhances skin quality. When selecting cheeses make sure they are rennetless (for easier digestion) and free from dyes or chemicals. Many adults do not handle dairy products (with the exception of butter) well, so use your discretion. However some people can handle goats or sheep's milk products more easily than cows milk derivations.

*Note that eggs are not considered a dairy product.

The following is a partial list:

Cheese, Cottage Cheese, Cream, Cream Cheese, Kefir, Milk, Yogurt

Food Combining Awareness for Healthy Digestion

If you are experiencing less than radiant health we have found that keeping the combinations of foods simple gives the body a chance to restore balance more easily. For some this may mean following these guidelines most of the time and for others maybe only one or two points will be necessary to maintain well-being. Much depends on your physical activity, lifestyle, reactions to life situations, age and season of the year as to what will work for you.

Please allow yourself to be flexible with your food choices as things change in your life, adapting the ideas in this book to suit your circumstances. Let your body be your guide in selecting what supports your individual needs at the time by utilizing the body feedback journal in this book. Your body will always tell you what can be handled.

• It is best to combine only one type of protein at a time per meal, ie. no eggs and steak (or breakfast meat), no cheese and meat, no eggs and cheese, no steak and shrimp, etc.

• When eating beef, lamb, liver, or veal, most people do well to avoid combining them with grains (rice, etc.), flour products (bread, chips, etc.) or starches (potatoes, etc.). This means avoiding hamburgers and french fries, lamb and potatoes, and beef and pasta. Beef, lamb, liver, veal and eggs also do not combine well with dairy products; this includes butter. When you eat red meat combine it only with low starch vegetables and nothing else (adding a small amount of oil to flavor is OK). This is a flexible point as some people when healthy do fine combining red meat with grains / flour products / vegetable starch.

• Wait at approximately 1 1/2 hours between meals and snacks.

• Wait at least 1 1/2 hours between eating vegetables and fruits. The only exceptions to this are lemons, limes and apples.

9

- Eat bananas alone and melons by themselves, as they are complex foods and may overload the system when combined with other foods.

- When eating chicken, turkey, fish or eggs, they combine well with grains, flour products, starchy vegetables and low starch vegetables for most people.

- Fruit, grains, flour products and diary will also combine fairly well.

- Protein can also combine with fruit.

Fats

All fats should be used sparingly, as they are a highly concentrated food and tend to congest the system if done to excess. Mayonnaise, butter (which is preferable to margarine), oils, coconut, avocado, nuts, nut and seed butters, and seeds all fall into this category. Read all labels carefully and be on the alert for hidden fats in packaged foods (i.e. breads, crackers, cookies, granola, and prepackaged cereals).

For adults in good health, 1 - 2 Tbls of added fat can be included daily if you eat animal protein, and 3 - 4 Tbls of added fat daily it you are vegan.

In the oil category, always buy cold-pressed oils and extra-virgin olive oil. Date all your oils, refrigerate, and discard them after 3 months,. Oils oxidize and become rancid when exposed to heat and/or light. When selecting a cooking oil, mono-unsaturated or high oleic oils are more molecularly stable than other oils at higher temperatures. Vary your intake of polyunsaturated oils as all provide a different balance of fatty acids to the body.

The following is a partial list:

> Butter, Mayonnaise, Nut Butters, Oils: extra virgin Olive ,Canola, Grape Seed, Safflower, Sunflower, Apricot Kernel, Hazelnut, Walnut, Flax, Pumpkin Seed (cold pressed oils are best).

Hydrogenated Fats and Oils like Shortenings and Margarine*

* The Age Accelerators

Trans Fatty Acids are formed when fats and oils are hydrogenated. During this process hydrogen molecules are added to polyunsaturated or monounsaturated oils, which then creates semisolid shortenings or margarines. The bad news here is that this modification makes the fat very difficult to digest. Furthermore many studies have now proven that these trans fatty acids unbalance the cholesterol in the blood which in turn leads to a variety of problems.

Salt

Fresh vegetables, proteins, grain and fruits provide all the natural sodium necessary for balance within the body. All forms of processed salt (i.e., sea salt, miso, tamari, and soy sauce) should be used with a very light hand and cooked into foods, not added at the table. It is best to use these condiments for special occasions, not daily use.

There are a number of reasons why salt in its inorganic crystalline form should be mostly avoided. First of all the fact that it is an inorganic compound and your body is designed to process only organic material, should give you a clue. Basically what excess salt does is cause the deterioration of your vital organs, especially the liver and the kidneys. It also interferes with the elimination of certain waste products of metabolism.

So why do we eat it and why are so many people hooked on it? Quite simply the answer is that it is a stimulant. In the same way that people use simple sugars, simple carbohydrates (flour) and caffeine, people use salt to give them a temporary energy boost because their nutrient poor, unbalanced eating habits are not giving them what they need. Unfortunately this short term stimulant strategy in the long run leads to all the ailments that we see in young and old alike today.

Fortunately, by reading and understanding this, you can act to change your habits and most likely avoid these problems. Here is a sobering figure that the U.S government and most scientists believe is true, that 75% of the disease in the U.S. is preventable and can be avoided through life-style/habit change.

So here is all you have to remember, your body needs organic sodium that is naturally found in vegetables (zucchini and other green low starch vegetables mostly), not processed sodium chloride in its crystalline forms of table salt or sea salt. Unrefined Celtic salt or Himlayan pink salt, which contain many beneficial minerals, may be an exception for some people if it is used occasionally and in very small amounts (1-2 pinches a day).

Caffeine

Caffeine intake should be moderated and in some cases eliminated. Not only does it deplete the body of many important "B" group vitamins, but it also may increase an individual's susceptibility to coronary heart disease, if so predisposed. Caffeine also hyper-stimulates the adrenal glands which over time can seriously deplete them. Coffee, black tea, diet sodas and most chocolates fall into this category. Think of using some of the many varieties of herbal teas available as a substitute. Green tea is not only very satisfying, but also stimulates the immune system, helps to reduce inflammation, balances blood sugar and calms the nervous system.

Concentrated Sugars

Refined sugars such as white sugar, molasses, corn syrup, and fructose, as well as all artificial sweeteners should be avoided. These have no nutritional value, providing only "empty" calories. Artificial sweeteners have also been implicated in many health problems.

Honey, agave, maple sugar, date sugar, barley-malt, rice-syrup, rice bran syrup, and fruit juice concentrates are very concentrated forms of naturally occurring sugars, so should be used in moderation.

For general use, in order of preference, try stevia, fruit juice concentrates, agave, rice syrup, rice bran syrup or powder, barley malt, maple sugar, date sugar, and finally, honey.

The wonderful exceptionally sweet tasting herb called Stevia can help with sweet cravings and does not raise blood sugar levels. It does not always do well in baking recipes but is quite good sprinkled on things or in drinks. It is highly concentrated so very little is needed for effect. It is also now conveniently available in a white powdered form in individual packets (just like artificial sweetener packets).

Alcohol

Like refined sugar, this substance also provides calories with minimal nutritional benefits and dehydrates the skin. Alcohol is even more rapidly converted in the body than refined sugar, reeking havoc with blood sugar levels, so use in moderation. Remember, when the liver and kidneys overload, the skin is the first part to show it.

Age Accelerating Additives - Glutamates

Glutamates are commonly found in the vast majority of prepared foods, even health food brands. Toxicologists point out that glutamates are neuro-toxins and are harmful to everyone. The following is a partial list of many types of glutamates:

> MSG, Accent, autolyzed yeast, ajinomoto, aspartame (acts like MSG), barley malt, malt extract, broth, bouillon, Chinese seasoning, carrageenan, calcium caseinate, disodium guanylate, disodium inosinate, dough conditioners, flavorings, natural flavorings (not all), flavors (i.e. turkey flavor), flutacyl, glutavene, gourmet powder, gelatin, hydrolyzed protein, hydrolyzed plant protein, hydrolyzed vegetable protein, hydrolyzed milk protein, kombu extract, L-Cysteine, monosodium glutamate, mono potassium glutamate, Mei-Jing, maltextrin, protein hydrolysate, RL-50, spices???, soy protein isolate, soy protein concentrate, soy sauce, Subu, sodium caseinate, smoke flavor, textured protein, vegetable broth, vegetable powder, vetsin, whipping agents, Wei-Jing, whey protein concentrate, protein isolate, yeast extract, zest.

> * Note: Artificial sweeteners such as aspartame, NutraSweet, Sweet and Low and Splenda are very harmful. It is better to eat sugar than to put these toxins into your system. Studies have shown that artificial sweeteners may shut down the production of leptin in the brain, which is the bio-chemical that signals when we are full.

Eating Out

Caution and questions are the keys to safe dining. Always ask if MSG is used, or sugar is added. Find out how the food is prepared and where it comes from. If the waitress of waiter is not sure, have them ask the chef. Also ask for sauces and dressings on the side. Most restaurants will accommodate you, especially if you have food sensitivities.

Where to Shop

Your local natural food store is by far the best place to shop. There are now natural food stores in just about every city and most larger towns. Your natural food store should carry foods that are not highly processed, organically grown produce and grains, and ethically raised, chemical free meats and poultry. Ethically raised means that the animals were not "factory farmed," or cruelly treated, and were fed a rich and healthy natural diet, instead of one full of junk, hormones and antibiotics. Chickens should be cage-free and their eggs should be fertile. Free range eggs are higher in omega fatty acids, as are free range beef and buffalo. It is beyond the scope of this book to delve deeply into the ethical, moral, and environmental issues of food. There are several excellent books available on these topics.

One common fallacy about natural food stores is that the food is often more expensive. Because a health supportive diet should include more fresh foods than processed foods, it costs less than the typical diet.

If you are not fortunate enough to live close to a natural food store you can also approach your local supermarket managers and ask them to carry the foods you would like to buy. Fortunately many major chains now have natural food sections and carry organic produce. Of course this is because customers such as yourself have asked for this.

Beware of health claims made on products from both health food and grocery stores. Claims such as "90% Fat Free," "No Preservatives," "No added sugar," "30% less calories," "Diet," "Sugar Free," etc., may mean very little for your health. A preservative free bread, for example, may have dough conditioners, sugar and added fat. A product with 30% less calories probably had 80% too many to begin with, and to cover up the lost flavor, may use other undesirable additives. Diet and Sugar Free products may have artificial sweeteners. Be a conscientious label reader. Otherwise, you'll never know what you're getting.

Some of the brands listed below may not be available at your local natural food store. These are brands that are available in most natural food stores, that we have found to be consistently good quality, without unnecessary additives. Other brands may be equally good. Just be sure to check the ingredients on the label. Remember they are listed in decreasing order of amount, so the predominant ingredient is listed first.

Simple Substitutions: Instead of . . .

Diet Sodas:

Perrier or mineral water with 1/2 glass of apple juice, white or purple grape juice, cranberry concentrate, or any of your favorite juices.

Pasta:

Soba (100% buckwheat), kamut, spelt, and rice pastas are a nice alternative to wheat based pastas (health food stores carry them in the oriental section). Rice noodles (available in health food stores), eggless noodles, Jerusalem artichoke noodles, eggless lasagna, fresh egg white based pasta.

Sweeteners:

Fruit juice concentrates (Hain and Bernard Jensen), Unsweetened frozen fruit juices (use full strength), pureed cooked or fresh, unsweetened frozen fruits. Amasake (a cultured rice product), barley or rice syrup (Yinnies, Mitoku, Sweet Cloud, Eden), Stevia (both liquid and powder).

Butter/Jams:

Unsweetened applesauce with or without cinnamon, homemade fruit purees or compotes, unsweetened or fruit juice sweetened preserves, (L.A., Sorrell Ridge, Westbrae, Poiret), unsweetened apple butter (L.A., Westbrae, Eden).

Non Yeasted Breads:

Corn tortillas, rice cakes (Lundbergs [the crunchiest], Hain, Chicosan, Pritikin), Lotus breads, Rudolphs all rye bread, Essene sprouted, unbaked at high heat breads (Essene, Garden of Eatin, Lifestream, Manna), mochi (pounded sweet rice cake). Mystic Lakes rice bread, Foods for Life rice bread. Pacific Bakeries or French Meadows kamut or spelt bagels and breads.

Sour Cream:

Lowfat yogurt mixed with herbs and spices.

Cheeses:

Rennetless, raw, low-fat, low or no sodium.

Milk on Cereals:

Soy milk. rice milk, oat milk, unsweetened coconut milk, nut milks, amasake, fruit juices.

Salad Dressing:

Try low oil or unsweetened health food brands.

Catsup/Tomato Sauce:

Try any of the health food store brands (Fruit juice sweetened, no salt is best).

Coffee Substitutes:

Emer-Gen C decafinated coffee with vitamins by Alacer, Cafe Roma, Caffix, grain based teas, Mugicha (roasted barley tea - health food store, oriental section), Dacopa, Creamy Carob herbal teas, Yogi teas, Decaf green tea.

Chocolate Substitutes:

Unsweetened carob powder, or unsweetened carob chips, candy bars, patties (rice, almond, or raisin crisps).

Mustard:

Low or no sodium mustard (natural food stores).

Cooking Wine:

Mirin (a Japanese liquid seasoning found in health food stores — Eden, Mitoku brands).

Ice Cream/Sherbets:

Rice Dream, Pure Decadence, So Delicious.

Waffles:

Van's oat bran with raisins, seven-grain. Rice flour waffles, wheat-free waffle mixes.

Cookies:

Mrs. Denson's, Pamelas and Barbaras brands all have wheat free and fruit juice sweetened recipes. Also try bread or toast with a little butter and fruit conserve or stevia powder and cinnamon.

Crackers:

Kalvi Crispbread, Wasa Rye, Wasa Lite Rye, Finn Crisps (the Wasa brand also has yeast free).

● *Diet / Low Fat Products*

Snack Foods Can = Accelerated Aging

*Note: Even if you are not overweight, this section still offers a lot of important information on how your body chemistry is negatively effected by many common foods.

With so many "Low Fat" snacks and foods available in the grocery stores, many people who are trying to manage their weight naturally are attracted to these items. This is because we have been led to believe that decreasing fat intake alone will lead to weight loss and good health. Unfortunately this has not proven to be true, as people continue to carry too much weight despite consuming ever greater quantities of low fat/diet foods.

While decreasing overall fat intake is a healthy approach, there are many other aspects of body chemistry that must be addressed in order to achieve lasting success. If you simply are replacing your favorite snack foods with low fat versions, then you can cause a weight gain even if your fat and calorie intake is lower than before.

To understand why this happens you need to realize how your body is designed to work. Over thousands of years our bodies have evolved to handle sugars as they are found in their natural whole forms, namely fruits, vegetables and whole grains (not flour products). Known as complex carbohydrates, these naturally sustaining foods are absorbed gradually into the blood stream with the help of a myriad of additional nutrients that are also present in the whole foods.

Simple sugars such as table sugar (sucrose), refined fructose, barley malt, maple syrup, honey, fruit juices, fruit sweeteners and refined simple carbohydrates (flour products, especially white flour, such as breads, cereals, pasta, noodles, cakes, cookies, rice cakes, etc.) rapidly raise blood sugar when ingested. When a rapid rise in blood sugar occurs the pancreas is triggered to release a hormone called insulin. The insulin in turn moves glucose (blood sugar) out of the blood stream and into the cells, thereby regulating the circulating blood sugar.

But because this response is not instantaneous, the pancreas continues to produce insulin even as the blood sugar is dropping from the initial simple sugar/insulin reaction. The unfortunate result of all this can be low blood sugar which tends to manifest as fatigue, foggy headed feeling, difficulty thinking, slow reaction and even aging skin.

Regrettably the reaction to the intake of the simple sugars does not stop there. In response to the drop in blood sugar, the adrenal glands begin to pump out greater quantities of the hormones adrenaline and cortisol. When your body does this it is using up precious stored energy. If this situation continues over a long period of time, the adrenals begin to wear down and conditions such as feeling chronically fatigued, anxiety and depression are the result. Also when insulin and cortisol levels are consistently high, cholesterol increases and the kidneys retain water and salt which in turn causes the blood pressure to rise. Repeated bio-chemical upsets stresses the entire immune system, contributing to more rapid aging.

As with the simple sugars, the simple carbohydrates (flour) produce the same results only at a slightly slower rate (considering that most snack foods are mostly a combination of flour, sugar and salt, you can see that this is a recipe for disaster. <u>I would like to point out here that even if you do not have a weight problem, eating too much simple sugars and carbohydrates can still adversely effect your immune system and accelerate the aging process.</u> This is especially important if you have immune related conditions such as allergies, asthma, chronic fatigue, fibromyalgia, lupus and other autoimmune processes including rheumatoid arthritis, irritable bowel syndrome or cancer.

Now here comes the part where the weight gain happens. Once your cells are saturated with all the glucose they can handle, the overflow is transformed into fat. Sometimes overweight people will develop a condition called "insulin resistance" which occurs when insulin is unable to move glucose into the cells. Here the cells keep sending the message for more glucose so the pancreas keeps on producing more insulin, but unfortunately the cells cannot accept any more. So a vicious cycle develops where the excess glucose is converted into fat and the more "low fat" products that you eat, the fatter you get. If this cycle is not corrected, chronically high blood sugar can result in type II diabetes.

OK, so what do I do to stop this from happening you ask? Fortunately the answer is quite simple; just treat your body as it was designed. And all that means is to eat well balanced whole foods in combination with moderate, regular exercise. Doing this will balance your blood sugar and when that happens you taking a big step toward better health.

Of course this is something that you may hear all the time, but you have not quite figured out exactly how to do it or maybe it seems too hard to do. Well that is where this book comes in handy because it is full of step by step specific guidelines. This book is also <u>not</u> about deprivation, but instead is a guide to help you find pleasure and health in foods that are truly good for you. Also I believe that exercise need not be a chore, but instead is something that can be fun.

Now the importance of exercise cannot be underestimated as its benefits are HUGE. First of all it produces chemicals in your brain that contribute to wellbeing, promotes sexual energy and helps you maintain a healthy weight. Although that sounds like enough of an enticement, here are also some specifics about how exercise promotes weight loss.

When you move your body in some form of gentle, sustained exercise for at least 15-20 minutes, glucose moves into your cells without the aid of insulin. This way your blood sugar stays balanced while your pancreas and adrenals get a rest. Also when your blood sugar is reduced during exercise, your insulin secretion is suppressed and your body uses stored glucose from the muscles and liver. This in turn results in the burning of more fat.

So with all this in mind, read on and explore all the ideas presented here that will help you balance your body and your life. I realize that what you are embarking on here may not be easy for you, so I have included a lot of information and ideas for you to choose from. Nothing in this book is extreme or harsh, everything here is designed to bring you gently into balance and harmony. So be kind to your self along the way and let this book guide you to a more healthy lifestyle.

● *Food Sensitivities*

Since this book is about helping you find what foods will work best for you, it can also be seen as a tool that will help you identify the foods that cause you problems. Just as the low fat / diet food problem is one mechanism that promotes poor health, there are others which we will put under the category of "food sensitivities."

Food sensitivities are a contributing factor to many people's health problems and are often a major cause of a depressed immune system. They are present or are developed for a number of reasons and even many natural whole foods can cause a reaction in a particular person. A depressed immune system also contributes to accelerated aging as well as many other health related issues.

One way people can develop food sensitivities over time is by eating a narrow diet and not rotating in a wide variety of foods. Many people are sensitive to such common foods as corn and wheat for this very reason, as they are common ingredients in just about everything a standard American diet (SAD) entails.

The other causes of food sensitivities are also mostly due to poor dietary habits and they include poor digestion, nutrient deficiencies, a limited diet of highly processed foods and very often "leaky gut syndrome" Leaky gut syndrome happens when the digestive tract is too permeable and allows toxins to enter the blood stream; this syndrome is often brought on by high alcohol consumption, the regular use of nonsteroidal anti-inflammatory drugs like aspirin, ibuprofen and acetaminophen, and assorted viral, bacterial, parasitic and yeast infections.

The following are some symptoms that people experiencing food sensitivities might exhibit:

> water retention, tending to gain several pounds in 1-2 days; trouble losing weight through restricting calories or exercising; losing weight while dieting but unable to get past a certain point; abnormal food cravings and binge eating; mental or physical fatigue and depression; puffiness or dark circles under the eyes; excess mucus or phlegm, chronically congested nose, runny nose or post nasal drip; poor digestion, bloating, flatulence, constipation alternating with diarrhea, nausea or abdominal pains/cramps; sore achy muscles or joints; frequent headaches; mood swings, irritability, panic attacks, hyperactivity, anxiety.

A common reaction for the food sensitive person is water retention. When partially digested food compounds pass through a compromised intestinal lining (leaky gut) into the bloodstream and eventually to the tissues, they cause irritation and inflammation. The body then attempts to reduce this irritation by diluting the offending material with fluid (note: practically all of my food sensitive clients experience immediate relief from this uncomfortable bloat when they follow the guidelines laid out in this book).

19

Food sensitivities can also cause problems through a process many of us are familiar with, namely food addictions. One study has found that partially digested compounds in food allergens act like morphine-like opiate drugs. This means that eating food allergens can cause a "high" that eventually wears off, thus producing a craving for more allergens in order to get back the euphoric sensation. By repeating this pattern people can become both physiologically and psychologically addicted. If a person tries eating less of these foods it's like asking an alcoholic to have one glass of wine a day. The cravings for these types of foods can become so uncontrollable that binge eating habits may develop.

Another point I want to emphasize here is that this information is not intended to replace the care and advice of medical professionals. I strongly urge you to seek the help of the qualified practitioners with whom you feel most comfortable; the information here will work well with any other treatment that you are following, consider it as a foundation for your health.

Currently there are two ways to determine what foods you are sensitive to. The first way is to have a blood test for food allergies. This method will give you some idea at that particular point of time as to what you might be allergic to. The downside of this approach is that your body's needs change hourly, daily and seasonally. So if you choose to do this, remember that it is only a "snap shot" but it will give you some guidelines.

The second way, and the one that ultimately works because it teaches body awareness, is to keep a body feedback journal (an example is provided in this book). Like a diary, you simply keep track of what you eat, when you eat it and how you feel. Another advantage this system has over the first, is that you can recognize and determine delayed reactions to foods; as much of the time a reaction may take as many as three days to surface. Also you can go back in the journal and see larger, seasonal patterns. And finally your doctor or other healthcare professional will find this information very useful.

* Note: A word about "gluten free"; Many people are sensitive to a particular gluten such as wheat or grains close wheat AND corn or soy itself. However many people may tolerate oats well even though oats are technically a gluten containing grain. So instead of avoiding all glutens, it may be a good idea to use the "Body Feedback Journal" to determine exactly which forms of gluten you react to. It is always best to try to eat the widest variety of foods possible in order to get the widest variety of nutrients.

● *Falling Off The Wagon*

One of the most frequent calls I receive is from guilt ridden clients who have "gone off" their diets. What I like to remind them of is that health supportive eating is a flexible rather than rigid approach that actually allows for life's celebrations and indulgences as well as for the inevitable back sliding into old self comforting patterns that is part of being human.

This a natural part of the process of balancing life with lifestyle that as you come more into harmony will happen less often. What occurs after you have been applying daily Jin Shin Jyutsu® self care and choose health supportive foods a good percentage of the time, is that the foods and activities that no longer serve your well being, will simply be something you are not attracted to anymore....or if you choose them occasionally, will not impact you as much .

For those times when you have eaten widely and feel poorly afterwards, having a cup of Bieler's Soup or lightly cooked low starch veggies every few hours for 1/2 to 1 day will help a lot. If you experience weakness or have low blood sugar, just have small amounts of protein with your Bieler's / veggies.

Applying some of the Jin Shin Jyutsu® self care flows as needed from "Self Help Book" 1 will also speed your recovery. Be gentle with yourself. The process of deep change may take some time and will go easier if you focus on acceptance rather than criticism.

● *A Word About Weight*

Each of us has an individual optimal weight that is easily maintained when eating an appropriate, varied whole foods diet combined with moderate, regular exercise It's important to remember that this "optimal" weight will vary as we age.

We are constantly bombarded with media generated images of young, exceptionally beautiful, very thin actors and models that most of the time have been liberally airbrushed, "Photo Shopped", and carefully staged to achieve the perfection they are trying to sell us. This can translate into unrealistic, unhealthy, and more importantly unattainable standards for women to compare themselves to.

While there is nothing wrong with wanting to make the most of what Nature has given you, trying to force yourself into a Madison Avenue or Hollywood ideal of beauty can make for a very unhappy life. Going for that number on a scale or waiting until you achieve the "perfect" clothing size in order to feel good about yourself only serves to deprive you of enjoying your life here and now. Instead think about your appearance as a creative canvas to have fun with expressing your one of a kind, unique beauty.

Over the years I have been in practice, I have seen a trend towards women getting pregnant for the first time into their mid forties. Many come to me because they experienced difficulties either in conceiving or carrying a child to term. After referring them to a medical specialist for a thorough assessment, I often found that these otherwise healthy women were simply too thin. After putting on 5-10 lbs. along with some lifestyle changes and appropriate Jin Shin Jyutsu® self care, many of these women would become pregnant within the year.

Certainly infertility and difficulty in carrying a child to full term can have many causes other than low body weight that need to be medically assessed..but if you have been given a clean bill of health and have been dieting for years and/or adhering to strenuous exercise programs in order to stay at your "target" weight, it may be a good idea to consider allowing yourself to gain a few pounds before trying to get pregnant.

Stringent dieting and exercising takes it's toll on your skin as well as your psyche no matter what age you are. Yo-yo dieting and low caloric intake can actually re-set your metabolic set point over time to require less and less calories. Once entrenched , this can be a difficult and frustrating cycle to turn around. As we age, we need to have a tad bit more body fat to ensure a smooth transition into menopause and beyond. Being rail thin OR carrying too much weight will imbalance the buffer women need as they approach 50.

Balance and moderation in all aspects of lifestyle choices is the key to optimal wellness as well as maintaining a youthful appearance throughout your life. Your body will tell you what your ideal weight is for the stage of life you are in, if you learn to listen. A Daily Body Feedback Journal is one of the simplest tools I have found to develop better "listening skills".

● *The Daily Body Feedback Journal*

Throughout this book we have given you tools to improve your health, vitality, well-being and slow the aging process. Since each of us is biochemically, and energetically unique, one way to find out which things work for us, make us feel and look better, and which things don't, is to keep a daily journal.

By keeping a journal you can learn a lot about how your body responds to different things. The journal is designed so you can keep a record of your daily food intake, your sleep, exercise, and stress patterns, your daily stool and urine output, as well as how you feel emotionally.

Through working with the journal you will become much more familiar with your body and how things affect it. Through this, you will learn what to do and what not to do, what to eat and what not to eat, and how to stay on top of things.

If you ever you begin to feel ill, or just not quite "right," the body feedback journal is a good way to point you in the right direction again. You may find that there is something new affecting you, or something that may not have affected you earlier is affecting you now. As we change, our bodies' needs also change.

The journal can be kept with you and filled out as you go, or you can do the whole day in the evening. Some people find it best to keep the journal with them through the day, for the first few weeks, then switch to morning and evening later on.

After you have a few weeks of journal compiled, you can go back over it and look for correlations. You might find that the day after you eat a particular food, you have gas, or feel constipated. If this happens every time you eat that food, it's a pretty good sign that this is a food you should avoid. Similarly, if you noticed on days that you exercised you had better bowel movements, or felt more energized, you know that is something you should continue to do. Look to both the physical and emotional symptoms as feedback for you to process.

The journals can be a very useful tool for your holistic health practitioner as well. He or she may be able to find patterns in your journal that you may not see right away. They can also gain a better sense of your life-style from your journal.

How to Use the Journal

Use a new page for each day. First note the date, the time you went to bed last night, and the time you rose this morning. You can then figure out how many hours you slept. Women should also note where they are in their menstrual cycle. If a woman is no longer cycling just note the correlations to the lunar cycle, as hormones ebb and flow in all species in relation to lunar cycles.

Your first entry should be about the quality of your sleep. Did you have uninterrupted sleep? Did you wake up during the night and when? Did you have nightmares? Next, Was it hard to get out of bed in the morning? Did you wake up with lots of energy or were you groggy? Then continue on as follows.

Use the journal to record any significant events through the day. Log in the foods you eat, liquids you drink, bowel movements, urination, exercise, a stressful or challenging situation, headaches, gas or other problems, medications or supplements you took (unless you take them every day) and treatments you receive. Note the time, and what you ate, drank and/or did. If it made you feel a particular way, write it down. If you feel a particular way half an hour later, start a new line, write down the time and how you felt.

Stay simple, just recording enough information for you to understand it. If you try to be too detailed, the journal can get to be too much trouble to keep up. It's important to make a commitment to keep the journal for at least one month, as many patterns may not reveal themselves in a shorter time. A sample journal page follows this section. You may copy the sample page for your own use.

Where Do I Start?

If you have read this far and have gone into your kitchen and looked at the ingredient labels of the foods that you have, there is a very good chance that most of the foods that you are eating regularly don't match the recommendations in this book. So where should you start?

Since the body feedback journal will work best if you can start from the basics, I suggest that you do your utmost to eat only the Bieler's vegetables (zucchini, green beans, celery, parsley) and protein (beef, chicken, etc.) for a few days. For most people this is a pleasant experience as they often lose a few pounds and experience more energy. Then as you feel like it, begin to add in <u>one at a time</u> small amount of grains, starchy vegetables, fruit and/or dairy. If you get a negative reaction such as a drop in energy, foggy head, bloating or just feel under par, go back to just the vegetables and protein

This is also the procedure that you should follow if you become sick. If you do this your illness will pass in a quarter of the time it would take otherwise. Also as you continue with your new eating plan you will detoxify more and more; and it is very likely that you will get to the point where you rarely get a cold or the flu. I personally have experienced this myself and I have also observed client after client getting to this point of optimal wellness.

Body Feedback Journal

Time	Food Eaten (What? How Much?)	Fluid Taken	Effect (physical - emotional)	Activity	Urination	Bowel Movement	Notes

● *Natural Supplements*

With 21st century hectic lifestyles, food choices and nutrient deficiencies in the soil our food is grown in, most of us need additional amounts of vitamins and minerals to stay healthy. Even though "natural" supplements are derived from natural sources, they are highly concentrated and processed. I feel it is best to view this category as "supplements to" rather than "substitutes for" a healthy diet and lifestyle. My preference is powders and liquids first and capsules second since there are usually less binders and fillers than are found in tablets.

The Staples

1) **A multi-vitamin** formulated for your age, activity levels, lifetsyle and sex that is easily absorbed in a bioavailable form.

2) **A multi-mineral** with 1:1 calcium and magnesium or with more magnesium than calcium in an easily absorbed, bio- available form.

Since many people have sensitivities to wheat, corn, soy , gluten and dairy, there are quite a few choices now available that are free of the above from the major natural food supplement companies.

If you are under stress, indulge frequently in sugar and/or alcohol, are experiencing sleep disturbances, or signs of hormonal imbalance, utilizing a formula with more magnesium than calcium can be a great support. Magnesium plays an important role in harmonizing the effects of our modern lifestyle. It activates close to 300 enzymes in the body and acts as a stress buffer by reducing the secretion of stress hormones. Magnesium can also quell sugar cravings, help to stabilize blood sugar, bolster cardio-vascular health, reduce inflammation in the body and help with PMS/peri-menopausal/menopausal symptoms. This important mineral also helps to regulate the mood enhancing hormone, serotonin. Most of us don't even come close to getting enough magnesium from our diets to maintain wellness.

3) **Vitamin D** (in the D3 form). Vitamin D3 is essential for calcium absorption promoting bone strength. It also reduces inflammation in the body and helps our immune system to function properly. Our body does have the ability to manufacture D3 naturally, but most of us don't get enough sun exposure especially during the winter months to give us what we need. Sunscreens which most of us use as protection from skin cancer block our bodies ability to make D from sunlight. Many MD's recommend 600-2,000 iu's daily. A simple blood test your doctor can order will pinpoint your individual needs.

4) Biosil - AKA orthosilic acid complex helps the body to regenerate collagen which declines with age. Along with enhancing collagen formation and skin elasticity, Biosil reduces fine lines and wrinkles, promotes healthy bones and joints, as well as strengthening nails and hair. Only a few drops a day are needed. Some sources recommend also using a pure hyaluronic acid supplement in addition to Biosil.

5) Vitamin E - Be sure to choose a natural form, preferably a mixed tocopherol blend in capsule form. Vitamin E is a powerful anti-oxidant which scavenges free radicals, protecting cells from oxidative damage. It's an important cardiovascular support as well as helping to keep skin youthful in appearance. Many MD's recommend 400-800 iu's per day. Caution must be used if you are taking blood thinners because vitamin E thins the blood.

6) Vitamin C is the premier anti-oxidant supplement which also supports collagen production and enhances the immune system. 500-1,000 mg. per day is what most sources recommend. Under periods of intense stress , you may require more. Bowel tolerance is the key factor here in determining how much to take.

7) Pro-biotics - Healthy elimination is critical to lovely skin. Pro-biotics are essential to balance the flora in our intestines and also supports our immune systems. Probiotics can be obtained from naturally fermented foods such as yogurt and kefir as well as the non-dairy sources of sauerkraut, fermented soy products like miso, natto and tempeh. You can also find pro-biotic supplements in the refrigerated section of most natural foods stores.

8) The Omega Family - The omega fatty acid group play a huge part in providing support for the cardio-vascular system, skin, central nervous and immune systems. They also contribute to hormonal balance, are nature's anti-inflammatories, improve mood, and cognitive functioning. I prefer to include omegas from a variety of food sources in my daily diet like freshly ground flax seed, refrigerated flax oils, nuts, seeds, vegetable oils and fish to provide a synergistically balanced spectrum of omegas. My favorite fish sources are sardines and wild caught salmon. Shoot for a balance of omega 3's (CLA, ALA, DHA and EPA) as well as the omega 6 and 9 fatty acids to complete your omega family needs. Caution: The omega's thin the blood and flax contains lignans which are a phyto-estrogen. So if you are taking blood thinners or have a predisposition to estrogen sensitive breast cancer, consult your doctor before ramping up your intake.

Some Resources To Explore

1) Pure Essence "Ionic Fizz" Cal+ with D and Mag+.

2) Peter Gillham's "Natural Calm"

3) Rainbow Light Women's and Men's Daily Vitamin and Calcium Plus Formula

4) Alacer "Emergen-C Lite"..easily portably with less sweeteners than the other formulas.

5) Jarrow Pro-biotics

6) Natural Factors "Biosil" and Jarrow "Biosil Formula"

7) Baxyl Hyaluronic Acid

In some cases, additional supplementation can be beneficial, so consult your holistic health care practitioner or MD. If you have questions.

● *Ageless Beauty At Your Fingertips*

The centuries old traditional Asian wellness art of Jin Shin Jyutsu® works with the body's subtle energy flows to restore and maintain physical harmony and mental-emotional balance. By gently holding specific locations in combination along these energy flow pathways you can facilitate the release of stress and tension as well as unlock your body's innate ability to heal naturally. Simply applying Jin Shin Jyutsu® self care on a daily basis keeps you literally in touch with your body's needs and signals, helping you to develop greater self awareness.

The benefits of Jin Shin Jyutsu® can be experienced as self care as well as from a trained Jin Shin Jyutsu® practitioner during private hands on sessions. Practitioners are also trained to offer basic self help classes and to design personalized self care as I do to support my client's individual needs. My personal Jin Shin Jyutsu® routines for general wellness and natural facial rejuvenation utilize the sequences outlined in Mary Burmeister's "Self Help Book 1" as the foundation with additional supplemental routines I have created for my individual needs. My opinion is that the sequences found in "Self Help Book 1" can be considered to be the cornerstone of any wellness and natural facial rejuvenation program.

I have found that by applying the "Trinity Flows" explained on pages 15-20 with the "Spleen Flow" found on (pages 39-42) before I get out of bed in the morning sets the tone for a wonderful day; and applying the "Main Central Vertical Flow"(pages 15-17) with the Stomach & Bladder Flows (pages 42-50) in the evening allow me to wind down and clear out the remnants of the day. During the day, I apply my additional personalized routines as time allows.

My overall health and resistance to stress has improved dramatically over the years I have employed the help of daily Jin Shin Jyutsu® self care with the bonus being a more youthful appearance. Friends I have not seen for years have remarked I now look younger and seem calmer than I did a decade ago.

Experiment to find the best combinations of Jin Shin Jyutsu® self care to suit your lifestyle.

Recommend Reading:

Jin Shin Jyutsu® "Self Help Books 1,2 & 3" by Mary Burmeister

"The Touch of Healing" by Alice Burmeister

All books available through www:JSJinc.net / (480)998-9331. List of practitioners throughout the world also available upon request.

The above notes were compiled from my understanding of Jin Shin Jyutsu® "Self Help Books 1, 2 & 3" as well as from the 5 Day Basic Jin Shin Jyutsu® seminars , special topic classes and self help classes I have taken. This material has been reviewed and approved by JSJ,Inc.

● *Stress Less*

Medical experts estimate that close to 90% of all disease processes are stress related or stress exacerbated. While we as humans don't experience the same stressors as our ancestors such as fleeing from wild animals or defending the village from invaders, our central nervous systems are the same. Modern unremitting stresses such as job worries, a volatile economy, and hectic schedules can have the same end effect.

When your mind perceives an event or ongoing events as a threat, your body interprets this perception as a "survival" situation shooting the hormone cortisol into your bloodstream which shuts down all but primary body functions to fight and flee. If this is a short term high stress situation like having a child dart in front of your car or a near miss auto accident, once the "threat" is removed, cortisol shuts down and the body begins to rebalance again. Unfortunately 21st century lifestyle and schedules often put our systems in a 24/7 survival mode which is damaging to all body functions.

Our reactions to perceived stressors also causes the body to produce a number of inflammatory chemicals in reaction to the cortisol release as well as suppressing many of the "feel good" brain hormones and slows the ability of our cells to repair and regenerate. This vicious cycle runs down the adrenals as well contributing to low energy, impaired immune systems and a host of medical labels such as fibromyalgia, EBV, Chronic Fatigue Syndrome, etc. that are so prevalent now. The chain reaction from chronically high cortisol levels is the root cause of many damaging processes in our body as well as contributing to the breakdown of collagen and elastin, thus prematurely aging us.

Some dermatologists also believe that the effects of chronic stress can weaken the skin's ability to act as a barrier to outside elements such as viruses, bacteria, and environmental pollutants. The impact of physical stressors such as illness, injury, poor diet, sleep deprivation, harsh weather, or even too much exercise all take the same toll on the body.

The good news is that taking a pro-active approach to bringing the body-mind out of "fight, flight, or freeze" can break this cycle and allow the body to re-balance itself. Simple tools you can use the moment you are aware of a stress triggered reaction like focusing on your breathing or just being aware that the response is happening can often nip it in the bud. Taking mindful short breathing breaks throughout the day when nothing challenging is happening can "build" your resistance to stress by giving you short spaces of relaxation. Regular stress reduction strategies such as taking walks in nature, doing yoga, praying, listening to relaxing music or applying the self care tools Jin Shin Jyutsu® provides, all also build in reserves of serenity to draw on when something challenging comes up. Anything that relaxes your body and mind releases the "feel good" brain chemicals and anti-inflammatory molecules that help to repair and regenerate you on all levels. Many other supportive strategies to reduce the impact of stress responses are offered throughout this book for you to explore.

Stress and Hormones

The production as well as the overall balance of all our hormones is critically impacted by chronic stress or periods of intense stress, whether that stress is mental / emotional or physical. As we age hormone levels fluctuate and eventually diminish, effecting skin quality, elasticity, and tone.

For women of all ages who are experiencing the effects of hormonal imbalance via the symptoms of PMS, post partum depression, peri-menopause, or menopause, there are many holistic approaches available to restore balance and reduce stress. Consulting with an herbalist, naturopath, or holistic health care practitioner who specialize in formulating herbs or nutritional supplements to address the root cause of your imbalance is one way to go. Regular acupuncture, acupressure, chiropractic, Jin Shin Jyutsu®, as well as other forms of body work can also be supportive to restoring harmony.

Bio-identical hormone therapy is another path many women of all ages are choosing to turn to . Bio-identical hormones are plant based formulations manufactured in labs or compounding pharmacies to be identical to those produced in the human body. There are many protocols and schools of thought on this subject, so I have included a few resources my clients have found helpful at the end of this section for you to explore. No one method works for all, so do your research, explore the many options and use your intuition to find what suits you.

Finally take time for yourself each day to just "be" without cell phones, TV, computer or schedules. It's amazing how just a few minutes of taking a time out can restore you on all levels. Making sure you have a strong emotional support system in place to be able to just simply connect and or vent when needed either by phone or in person also goes a long way to creating well being. We are social creatures who absolutely need to feel connected to others who love and care about us as we do them or our psyche and our physical health suffers.

Epsom Salt Bath and Foot Soaks

One of my favorite daily "time outs" is a 20 minute soak in a warm epsom salt bath with equal amounts of unprocessed sea salt infused with essentials oils. The tensions and aches of the day literally float away! From ancient times, natural hot springs pools have been recognized for their restorative properties. Epsom salt baths and foot baths are the "at home" version of this time honored practice. This compound is formed naturally from evaporated brine pools in the earth's crust and is composed of magnesium and sulfates . Epsom salts are easily absorbed through the skin reducing inflammation, soothing sore muscles, and flushing toxins from the body while enhancing total mind-body relaxation.

I use 2 cups of Epsom salts to a warm to hot bath and soak for 15-20 minutes. For a foot bath, add 1 cup to your soaking container of warm to hot water and relax for 15-20 minutes. The addition of any favorite essential oils amplifies the experience. For an alternative therapeutic soak, add equal amounts of natural sea salts such as Dead Sea or Himalayan to your epsom bath or foot bath.

Make sure to use pure, USP Food Grade epsom salts for soaking.

Caution: If you have high blood pressure or any other medical condition, consult your medical doctor before using epsom/sea salt soaks.

Here are some resources to explore:

Salt Works
Ultra Epsom Salts/ Himalayan / Dead Sea Bath Salts
www:seasalt.com (800) 353-7258

San Francisco Bath Salt Company
www:sfbsc.com
(800) 480-4540

Young Living Oils- essential oils of high quality
www:youngliving.com

Jin Shin Jyutsu® self help books and practitioners
www:jsjinc.net
(480) 998-9331

Virginia Hopkins Newsletter
a free online newsletter on bio-identical hormones therapy and test kits
www:virginiahopkinstestkits.com
(888) 438-1211

Women's International Pharmacy
economically priced , high quality compounding pharmacy that ships throughout the US.
www:womensinternational.com
(800) 279-5708

HM Enterprises
over the counter bio-identical hormone source
www:hmenterprises.com
(800) 742-4773

● *Sleep . . How To Get Your Beauty Sleep*

Good quality and appropriate amount of sleep is critically important to maintaining optimal health and keeping a youthful appearance. It is during the deep phases of sleep that our bodies regenerate and our minds rest. Chronic "under sleeping", sleep deprivation, or simply lack of good quality sleep raises stress hormone levels which cause the breakdown of collagen and our cells ability to repair.

Here are a few general tips to set the stage for a good night's rest:

1) Limit caffeine intake after 3pm.

2) Avoid sugary snacks, but especially close to bedtime as they negatively impact blood sugar.

3) If you take B vitamins, take them before the mid afternoon as they can disrupt sleep patterns.

4) Do your cardio or other forms of vigorous exercise early in the day, focusing on more relaxing activities like yoga, Tai Qi, Qi Gong, or Feldenkrais closer to bedtime.

5) Avoid alcohol close to bedtime because it can cause sleep disruption and dehydration even though the initial effect is relaxing.

6) Keep a notebook by the bed to pen your concerns or "to do's" to be addressed the next day rather than running them around in your head all night.

7) Make your evening meal a light one to avoid going to bed overfull. See the Diet section for recipe ideas.

8) Find some tools to reduce daytime stress and to unwind with at night. See Stress Less, Ageless Beauty At Your Fingertips And The Inner Connection sections for ideas.

9) Sleeping in a cool room with temps under 69F can enhance both sleep quality and the ability to stay asleep.

10) If you have issues either staying asleep or falling asleep due to sound sensitivity, many of my clients have found using earplugs or a white noise machine helps them tremendously.

11) For women who experience insomnia before periods or during peri-menopause/menopause, help in balancing hormones can greatly assist in restoring sleep patterns. See the "Stress Less" section for resources.

12) Finally shooting for 6-8 hours of uninterrupted sleep on a regular basis lays a good foundation for optimal wellness and a youthful appearance.

Timing Is Everything

It is important to remember that all living creatures animal and human have bio-rhythms that are influenced by the cycles in nature. The monthly magnetic tidal pulls of the sun and the moon, seasonal and diurnal temperature variations, seasonal light fluctuations, as well as the cycles of light and darkness during a 24 hour period all effect the functioning of our circadian rhythms. The seed of many disease processes lie in living out of sync with these rhythms of nature. The impact of light and darkness on sleep quality is what I will explain next.

The timing of actual lights out and exposure to artificial light after nightfall plays a very important role in getting a good night's sleep. Your brain releases the sleep inducing hormone melatonin in response to darkness increasing between 9 and 11pm. Since this is the hormone that lulls us into sleep allowing our bodies to work on cellular repair and regeneration, it's important to dim the lights or have a total lights out close to 9pm.

Another point to address is that many people go to bed with bright lights on until just before sleep, fall asleep in front of the TV, or sleep in a room bathed in ambient light from either outside artificial light or from the many LED's that beam from home electronics like alarm clocks, dvd players, TV etc. These factors can interfere not only with how quickly you fall asleep, but how deeply you sleep, how interrupted your sleep cycle is, and when you wake up.

Bright artificial light after sunset is unnatural throwing both our circadian rhythms and our hormones out of wack. Some recent studies have shown that regular exposure to bright artificial light after nightfall and ambient artificial light after nightfall increases the risk of breast cancer, depression, anxiety, suppresses the immune system, and even contributes to weight gain.

Some simple strategies are to turn down the lights after sunset using low wattage incandescent bulbs or candlelight, lowering the brightness setting on your computer monitor, and working towards TV off by 10pm. Make sure to turn off or cover as many LED's from bedroom electronics before 9pm. Instead of watching TV right up until lights out, TIVO or record your favorite programs and perhaps read a favorite book in comfortably dim light until sleepy. Make sure that if you need to get up during the night to avoid getting a blast of bright light from opening the refrigerator door or turning on a bedside lamp. Motion sensitive dim night lights that simulate moonlight can be strategically placed in your bathroom and hallway help to keep you safe from falls while making it easier to drift back into a deep sleep. Even a short burst of intense light at night can interrupt the hormonal production needed to allow deep states of sleep. Some people are so sensitive to blasts of light from outside like headlights or the neighbor's motion sensitive security lights that black out curtains are a must. This is particularly so for women going through peri-menopause or menopause because of the hormonal fluctuations.

● *Exercise . . . Move It Or Lose It*

Human beings are meant to move. When we don't get the appropriate amount of regular movement, the risk of just about every known ailment increases as well as accelerating the aging process. Balanced activity strengthens the immune system, boosts your metabolism, lifts mood, increases energy, helps to stabilize blood sugar, and reduces stress. Regular moderate exercise also reduces muscle and bone loss and strengthens muscles including your most important muscle, your heart.

One of the perks is that your appearance is improved by toning your body, posture is enhanced and your skin receives a healthy glow due to the increased circulation regular exercise provides. In a nutshell, a moderate, diverse exercise plan is a crucial component in slowing the aging process and creating optimal health for a lifetime.

A balanced movement program needs to include regular forms of moderate aerobic exercise and strengthening routines, as well as some form of what I call meditative movement. In the aerobic category, just 20 minutes, 3-4 times a week will fill the bill. Walking, hiking, tennis ,cycling, dancing, swimming, roller skating , and horseback riding can all be forms of aerobic exercise. Setting up a stationary bike or mini trampoline in front of the TV or going window shopping in an indoor mall can be an easy winter time way of getting your aerobic quotient.

Pilates, Bar Method, or some types of yoga either with DVD's or classes, weight or resistance training plans are some of the many choices available to help integrate the strength training module into your life. Many people find that making an exercise "date" with friends to either go to class or have your own class watching a DVD at home helps to keep them on track. Just 30 minutes 2-3 times a week is adequate.

Meditative movement forms such as the gentler types of yoga, Qi Gong, Tai Qi, Feldenkrais or even gardening can benefit the body and mind in a slightly different way, by helping to relieve stress, calm and center the mind, and promote a balanced energy flow throughout the body.

When to exercise can be a challenge for many people. By choosing a regular time and schedule, it will be much easier to be consistent. Some people feel best exercising in the morning because it gives them an invigorating start to the day, while others find exercising in the early evening helps them unwind from a stressful day. Try to get some of your exercise outdoors whenever possible to connect with one of our greatest healing resources...Nature. Remember to choose activities that are enjoyable and can be easily incorporated into your lifestyle on a continuing basis.

Resources To Explore:

Balanced Body - a great resource for Pilates books, DVD's, and certified practitioners
www:balancedbody.com (800)745-2837

Feldenkrais Method - downloads and CD's of Feldenkrais Awareness Through Movement sequences. www:feldenkraisathome.com /(310)470-6483.

● *The Inner Connection -*
Beauty Is More Than Skin Deep

Ageless beauty is much more than just the appearance of the physical form. It's a mirror of the connection to a deeper state that many spiritual traditions call our True Self, Soul, or Essence.

Each of us is a totally unique expression of Source with valuable gifts to contribute to those around us. I believe that we have a dual purpose during our time on earth, an inner purpose which is connecting to our Essence and an outer purpose which is an expression of our unique gifts as well as the vehicle for bringing forth our True Self into this world.

When you fulfill your inner purpose, you are then an expression of that Self in whatever life situation you find yourself in. Your outer purpose, what you do to make money, who you marry, what you do for fun, becomes the vehicle for Creator to express through you. Through societal, cultural, and familial conditioning so many of us get stuck in counterfeit responses to life situations that are not the real "us". Once you are consistently able to connect with Source, all these layers will simply fall away, leaving the True You to shine through.

Regular quiet time alone is essential to establishing a strong connection to your inner Self. It's like building a muscle. When you connect regularly to your Self which is connected to Source, that sense of peace and calm stays with you to draw upon even in life's inevitable challenging situations. Whenever you are able to still your mind, be it through mini conscious breathing breaks throughout the day or via a more structured meditation practice, you open a space for your True Self to come forth. If you are totally immersed, present in any activity you do, you access this immense power. Walking in nature, meditation, gardening, prayer, guided imagery tapes, the ancient harmonizing art of Jin Shin Jyutsu®, or just listening to your favorite music all can facilitate inner connection as can any of your daily activities if done with total focus.

Finding an outlet for your creativity is another wonderful access point to peace. Whenever you do something you love with all your heart, the mind is stilled and peace emerges. Journaling, sculpting, making jewelry, decorating, cooking or playing a musical instrument can all be access points to stillness when they are done with presence

Here is a resource that offers many different approaches to connect with your Inner Self:

Sounds True Inc.
413 S. Arthur Ave.
Louisville, CO 80027
(800) 333-9185 or (303) 665-3151
www:soundstrue.com / info@soundstrue.com

● *Natural Skin Care Basics*

A regular daily natural skin care regime is an essential part of creating healthy skin and a youthful appearance. The basic program would include selecting a daily cleanser, toner and hydrator appropriate for your age, skin type, climate you live in, the season of the year, as well as additional products to target specific needs. These additional products could include a serum as well as weekly intensive products such as peels, masks, and exfoliators.

Since each of us is unique, with specific skin care needs, consulting with a professional esthetician who specializes in natural skin care can be of great help in selecting products that will compliment you as an individual. Regular facials deep cleanse your skin and can provide a more intensive peel, exfoliator, mask or specialized treatment than you can use safely at home. They are also a super way to just relax and allow yourself to be pampered.

Please note that many products labeled as moisturizers, "natural" or not, are formulated with heavy, pore clogging ingredients that do not penetrate the skin's layers simply sitting on top of the skin. They may temporarily make the skin feel softer, but since they do not allow the skin to breathe can create long term issues such as enlarged pores, blackheads, and lead to decreased skin elasticity due to lack of proper oxygenation. This is where a natural skin care professional can be of service to you, pointing you to the line or lines that fit your needs and budget.

Some form of UV protection in the form of a sunscreen SPF 15 or higher is a must to prevent visible aging of the skin , hyperpigmentation and most importantly skin cancer. Sunscreen is the most effective topical defense against premature aging of the skin you can use. Make sure you protect all exposed areas of the skin. Many people concentrate on applying sunscreen to the face and front of the neck, forgetting to protect the delicate chest area, back of the neck, ears, and hands. A stylish wide brimmed hat goes along way to provide additional sun protection.

One of the simplest anti-agers you can add to your toolbox is to invest in a set of pure silk pillow cases. We all spend at least 6-8 hours a day for our entire lives sleeping. The repeated weight of your head pushing your face against a pillow case that grabs the skin or bunches up will create "sleep creases" that don't disappear over time and will actually worsen existing lines. The slippery texture of natural silk pillow cases allows your skin and hair to glide over the surface when you change positions during the night making for more restful sleep and reduces skin drag. This luxurious addition also keeps your head and face cooler which can help induce deeper sleep states.. And best of all you wake up free of the dreaded "bed head".

Skin Exposure - Ingredients To Limit

Your skin is the largest organ in your body and is also part of your "intake system". This means that whatever you come into physical contact with can enter your system via your skin because skin is permeable. So it makes sense to be as careful as possible in this category as you are with what goes into your mouth. Choosing products that are free of toxic ingredients also protect our earth. Whatever you put on you skin eventually gets washed down your drain and into our waterways.

Deodorants and toothpastes are an additional category of daily use personal care products that also need to be chosen with care to avoid or minimize toxic ingredients. The armpit and inner mouth areas rapidly deliver any substance used topically into your blood stream, so make your choices health enhancing ones whenever possible.

All that being said, I have found it to be nearly impossible to eliminate all questionable ingredients in the makeup and hair styling product categories. Many "all natural" cosmetic and hair styling products either don't perform as well as the "leaded" variety or include natural ingredients I am sensitive to. It's important to remember that just because an ingredient is "natural" does not mean you can not have a reaction to it. So I choose my "leaded" products carefully making sure I both limit the amounts and number I use on a daily basis choosing "toxic chemical free" whenever possible. Life is a balancing act, so do your homework and choose wisely for your needs. Cruelty free/non-animal tested is the category that I do not compromise on and choose 100% of the time because it is not necessary to subject animals to any pain or cruelty in order to test products for human use.

The following is a list of the top toxic ingredients I recommend my clients limit or avoid when possible:

DEA (diethonelamine), MEA (monoethanolamine, TEA (triethnolamine), DMDM Hydantoin and Urea (Imidazolidinyl), F,D and C Color Pigments , Synthetic Fragrances, Mineral Oil, Polyethylene Glycol (PEG), Propylene Glycol (PG) and Butylene Glycol, Sodium Lauryl Sulfate (SLS) and Sodium Laureth Sulfate (SLES), Parabens.

Here are some of my favorite resources:

1) Arcona Skin Care Products
The Arcona Studio
425 Broadway, Suite B
Santa Monica, CA 94041
www.arcona.com (877) 272-6620
info@arcona.com

2) Mychelle Natural Dermaceuticals
www:Mychelle.com (800)447-2076

3) Nonie Of Beverly Hills: Natural skin care products for women and men
www:nonieofbeverlyhills.com (888)666-4324

4) Home Health's Rosewater or Lavenderwater Bath Splash and Perfume
www:homehealthUS.com (800)445-7137

5) Naturally Fresh Deodorant Crystal Spray
www:tccd.com

6) Crystal Deodorant Spray
www:thecrystal.com

7) Association of Holistic Skin Care Practitioner's
www:holisticskincarepractioners.org

Cosmetics I love

Senna Cosmetics - although not a 100% "natural" line of boutique makeup, their products are what I have used since 1986 because I have no negative reactions to most of their cosmetics and I adore the natural look they offer. Their line offers a wide range of fashion forward color choices for all ethnic groups, the quality is superb, and they are economically priced. Eugenia Weston, the owner, also made her entire line 100% non-animal tested and cruelty free from the time she opened her doors, before it became fashionable to do so. If you are ever in the LA area, make sure to schedule an appointment with Eugenia for a makeup consult. In my opinion, she has one of the best set of eyes in the business specializing in creating natural, age appropriate color palettes designed to enhance your own unique beauty. They are available online or through any of the Senna Boutiques in the greater Los Angeles area. www:sennacosmetics.com / (800) 537-3662.

● *Other Lifestyle Factors*

Smoking Cigarettes

Of course we all know that smoking is not good for anyone, but we also know that nicotine is one of the hardest addictions to overcome. Smoking accelerates the breakdown of collagen and elastin which are the structural proteins that give skin its youthful appeal. Also second hand smoke can impact your health and well being so avoid being around smokers for extended periods of time whenever possible.

Fortunately there are a number of effective methods that can help ease the process such as acupuncture, Jin Shin Jyutsu® and hypnosis. So with that in mind I would like to present some "positive" motivational information that will help you realize the specific benefits of quitting. It is never too late!

Quitting smoking is the single greatest thing you can do to improve your health.

When smokers quit, within <u>20 minutes of smoking that last cigarette</u>, the body begins a series of changes that continue for years:

<u>20 minutes</u> - blood pressure drops to normal, body temperature of hands and feet increases to normal, pulse rate drops to normal

<u>8 hours </u>- carbon monoxide level in blood drops to normal, oxygen level in blood increase to normal

<u>24 hours</u> - chance of heart attack decreases

<u>48 hours</u> - nerve endings start regrowing, the ability to smell and taste is enhanced

<u>2 weeks to 3 months</u> - circulation improves, walking becomes easier, lung function increases up to 30 %

<u>1 to 9 months </u>- coughing, sinus congestion, fatigue, shortness of breath decreases, cilia regrow in lungs, increasing the ability to handle mucus, clean the lungs and reduce infection

<u>1 year</u> - excess risk of heart disease is half that of a smoker

<u>5 years</u> - lung cancer death rate for average smoker (1 pack a day) decreases by half, stroke risk is reduced to that of a nonsmoker 5-15 years after quitting, risk of cancer of the mouth, throat, esophagus is half that of a smoker

<u>10 years</u> - lung cancer death rate similar to that of a nonsmoker, precancerous cells are replaced, risk of cancer of the mouth, throat, esophagus, bladder, kidney and pancreas decreases

<u>15 years</u> - risk of coronary heart disease is that of a nonsmoker

Some Basic Tools for Quitting

Stay in the moment. When a life situation triggers you acknowledge that trigger and do some Jin Shin Jyutsu® self care or take a walk to reconnect to your body.

Take a breather, literally, a few conscious breaths while doing self help Jin shin Jyutsu® can head off most cravings. Relaxation exercise like yoga and Qigong help relieve urges to smoke; remember that urges to smoke are temporary, stay in the moment!

Exercise, especially moderate aerobic exercise like walking, bicycling and swimming will help relieve tension and your urge to smoke

Quitting Tips

Enjoy nibbling on items like carrots, celery or apples, or suck on cinnamon sticks

Stretch out your meals, pause between bites

After dinner, instead of a cigarette, treat yourself to a mint or a cup of herb tea

Other Lifestyle Factors

Exposure to Human Made EMF

Human made Electrical Magnetic Frequencies (EMF) are all around us, especially those of us who live in dense urban areas. Science is trying to determine exactly how EMF affects humans but it is generally conceded that too much EMF is quite harmful to any living organic being. At its very worse it may promote cancer and at its least it can be a stress producing irritant. Recent research indicates that high levels of EMF may also interfere with melatonin production which negatively impacts sleep as well as your immune system.

Human made EMF has many sources which include CRT's (cathode ray tubes. ie. computer monitors, TV's), microwaves, cell phones, fluorescent lights, power lines, etc. Since these are common and useful fixtures of modern life, completely eliminating them would not work for most people. Fortunately if precautions are taken, most people can minimize the negative effects of these things.

So how can you protect yourself from human made EMF? Well the simplest and most effective tool is to limit your exposure. The most obvious way to do this is to not spend a lot of time using or in the proximity of these devices. Secondly, when you do use EMF emitting appliances, keep a good distance between you and it (ie. don't stand right next to the microwave). Fortunately most EMF generated by appliances dissipates rapidly beyond 2-3 feet. So some other good strategies here are to watch TV from across the room, place your computer monitor at the far end of the desk and put your computer on the other side of the room (you can usually run about 8 ft. of cable extensions without loss of monitor clarity).

That sounds like some good advice you might say, but what if I have to work in environment with a lot of computers and other equipment? Well first of all there are some things like monitor screens that may help, but primarily I would recommend getting some nifty little personal EMF protection devices from The Energy Works (email: energyworks@earthlink.net website: http://www.energy-works.net). These handy things can be worn or placed in your environment to effectively neutralize human made EMF.

● *Putting It All Together*

Making lifestyle changes that will serve you for the long haul involves a patient, systematic approach.

Think about selecting the easiest areas for you to integrate first, maybe picking a few ideas a month from each section to try if starting the entire program seems overwhelming. If you backslide or don't do everything "just right", know that by even making a few of the changes suggested here as part of your daily routine, you will make a huge impact on the overall quality of your life, with the bonus being a more youthful appearance.

Remember somewhere around 30 days after adding any change to your daily routines, it becomes a habit. You can then move on to implementing the next step or steps . If you incorporate 1-2 ideas a month from the entire program, in one year you will have a whole new you.

As the ancient proverb says, " A journey of a thousand miles begins with one step". Enjoy the process, be kind to yourself, and make it your own for a lifetime.

● *Simply Delicious Recipes*

Quick and Easy Cooking Suggestions

● Borrow a tip from the Asia and wrap an occasional meal in a leaf of lettuce. Spread the lettuce leaf with some low/no sodium mustard and top with sliced or shredded chicken, turkey, salmon, tuna or steamed veggies hot/cold.

● Save cooked leftover veggies and toss with chilled cooked brown rice, shredded lettuce and chilled steamed veggies. Toss lightly with your favorite dressing.

● Steam your favorite veggies with onions or leeks until tender and puree in a blender with a little mirin and herbs for a creamy soup.

● Stretch sauces with chicken stock or lemon juice, not oil or butter.

● Use steamed vegetable water as a base for stocks and sauces.

● Stretch small amounts of fish and chicken by serving on a colorful bed of shredded or julienned cabbage, carrots, zucchini, summer squash, etc., steamed with herbs until tender, crisp.

● Use pureed vegetables to thicken sauces and soups.

● Use lemon juice, not oil, to prevent sticking when cooking pasta.

● Puree carotene rich veggies (orange/yellow colored) with a little cooking water for use in breads and muffins. Best suggestions are: carrots, pumpkin, winter squashes, yams, sweet potatoes.

● Chop your favorite ripe fresh fruits and layer with plain yogurt for a healthy dessert parfait.

● Use a few drops of oil with herbs over baked yams/sweet potatoes / pastas. Toasted sesame oil is particularly tasty!

● Toss 1 Tbls. of sunflower/sesame/pumpkin seeds or pine nuts into your cooked rice for a little extra crunch. Cooked chestnuts are also quite good.

Trimming the Fat (But Not The Flavor!)

Acceptable Cooking Fats (may also be used for non-heated uses):

> Unsalted raw butter
> Olive Oil (extra virgin or virgin only)
> Sesame Oil (toasted or plain)
> Canola (health food only)

Acceptable Oils for Non-Heated Uses (Cold-Pressed Only):

Safflower	Avocado	Almond	Hazelnut
Flax	Sunflower	Walnut	Pecan

Date all oil when purchased, store in the refrigerator and discard after three months. For optimum health, oil intake should not exceed two Tablespoons daily. Always choose 100% cold expeller pressed oils.

If you choose to include cheeses (raw, rennetless only please) and/or nut butters (unsalted, no hydrogenated fats or sugars) be aware that these are concentrated fats, so adjust your oil intake accordingly.

Most Desirable Cooking Techniques:

Steam	Bake	Grill
Poach	Stew	Roast
Broil	Water-Saute	Blanch

A swipe of oil or butter can be used for flavor in water saute. When blanching, dip veggies in boiling water for a short time.

Stir Fry (for occasional use only) with 1 Tbls. oil, plus chicken/vegetable stock to prevent sticking.

Oil may be tossed into cooked veggies after cooking with a few herbs or spices for flavor. Place oil in small plant mister bottle. Spray on salads, coat a pan for sauteing, or over steamed veggies for a more even coverage with less oil.

Cereal and Grain Dishes

• Rice Pilaf

>   1 cup long-grain brown rice
>   2 cups water
>   2 Tbls. mirin
>   2 Tbls. butter
>   2 large bay leaves
> $1/8$ tsp. white pepper
>   2 Tbls. chicken stock
> $1/2$ cup diced green peppers
> $1/2$ cup diced onions
> $1/2$ diced mushrooms

Combine ingredients except rice and veggies in $1 1/2$ quart saucepan. Bring to a boil. Add rice, cover, turn flame down and simmer for 20 minutes. Stir in vegetables and continue simmering until tender (about 15 minutes). Stir occasionally. Turn off heat and allow to sit covered 10-15 minutes. Fluff with fork, and serve.

• Millet "Mashed Potatoes"

> $2 1/2$ cups water
>   1 garlic clove, minced
>   1 onion, minced
>   2 Tbls. vegetable oil
> $1 1/4$ cups cauliflower pieces
>   1 cup millet
>   Freshly ground pepper, to taste

In a large saucepan, saute the garlic and onion in the oil over moderate heat for 5 minutes, until softened. Add the cauliflower, millet and $2 1/2$ cups of water. Cover and cook over low heat for 20 minutes.

In a blender or food processor, puree until smooth. Keep warm in a covered saucepan until ready to eat. Serve with Miso Mushroom Gravy (p.61).

• Home Made Flour (Millet, Rice, Oat)

To make your own fresh flour from any of the above grains simply grind the grain in a coffee grinder or regular blender until powdered. Any of these flours may be substituted for wheat flour in a recipe. Just make sure to add $1/2$ tsp. more of low sodium baking powder than the original recipe calls for.

• Savory Biscuits

> 2 cups millet/rice/oat flour
> 1 1/2 Tbls. low sodium baking powder
> 1 Tbls. dill weed
> 1/2 tsp. garlic powder
> 2 fertile eggs, well beaten
> 2 Tbls. unsalted butter

Sift all dry ingredients together. Add eggs and melted butter to form a very stiff dough. If batter is too stiff to handle add a few drops of water. Drop by Tbls. onto a lightly greased baking sheet and bake at 325 degrees for 15 to 20 minutes.

• French Toast

> 2 slices bread (whole grain)
> 2 fertile eggs, well beaten or 2 egg whites & 1 Tbls. water
> 2 tsp. cinnamon
> 1 tsp. vanilla extract
> 1 Tbls. water
> 1 Tbls. unsalted butter, melted

Melt butter in a skillet. Blend liquids, eggs, and spices and soak bread until saturated. Brown in skillet on each side and place under broiler to toast briefly. Top with Fruit Compote (see recipe) and/or yogurt.

• Millet Pilaf

> 2 cups cooked millet
> 1 onion, finely chopped
> 1 med. tomato, chopped
> 1 small apple, peeled and diced
> 1 tsp. rosemary
> 1/2 tsp. garlic powder or 1 clove, finely chopped
> 1/2 tsp. cayenne pepper
> 1/2 cup apple juice, unsweetened
> 1/2 tsp. curry powder
> 1/2 tsp. basil
> 2 Tbls. unsalted butter

Melt butter in a skillet and add onions, garlic, herbs, and spices. Saute until onions are transparent. Add apples and juice and saute for an additional 3 to 5 minutes. Stir in millet and tomatoes and cook for 3 to 5 minutes. This may also be used as a delicious stuffing for Cornish game hens, chicken or turkey.

• Five Minute Breakfast - Grain Custard

1 large fertile egg
1/4 cup plain or vanilla-pecan amasake or rice/oat milk
1/2 cup cooked grain (brown rice, millet, quinoa, barley, oat groats, kasha, rye berries) or
1/2 cup quick cooking cereal (cream of rye, cream of rice and rye, oatmeal, oat bran)
1/2 tsp. no-sugar vanilla extract
1/2 tsp. cinnamon

Place egg, amasake, vanilla and cinnamon in a blender and whip well. Pour egg mixture into the quick cookinginto a custard-like consistency. Serve immediately topped with fresh fruit, fruit compote, fruit juice sweetened conserves, raisins, or plain.

• Hot Cereal

1 cup raw oats/millet/rye/quinoa/amaranth
1 cup water

Cook over low heat until done (rye/oat groats 20-25 minutes, amaranth/millet/quinoa 25-30 minutes).

Toppings: R.W. Knudsen coconut nectar/unsweetened applesauce with cinnamon/chopped fresh fruit/un-sweetened fruit jams or butters/amasake/Fruit Compote (see recipe).

• No Flour Pancakes

1 cup cooked millet, rice, rye, oats, or mixtures
1 fertile egg
1/4 to 1/2 cup any fruit puree/applesauce

Mix all ingredients in a blender. Drop by spoonful onto a hot nonstick skillet. Cook until lightly browned on both sides. Serve topped with your favorite fruit puree or syrup (a few chopped nuts or seeds may be added to the batter if desired).

47

● Summer Pasta Salad

    2 cups cooked pasta (Kamut, Soba, Rice or Wheat)
    1 - 8 oz. pkg. frozen peas
    2 cups fresh broccoli flowerettes
    3 cloves garlic, minced
    3 Tbls. parsley, finely chopped
    2 Tbls. olive oil
    2 Tbls. mirin
    2 Tbls. fresh basil, finely chopped

Saute broccoli and garlic in olive oil until just tender adding water to prevent sticking. Then add frozen peas and mirin, cover and simmer 5 to 8 minutes. Add parsley and basil and toss briefly with existing veggies. Remove from heat and toss well with pasta. Chill at least one hour and serve cold or at room temperature.

● Vegetable Couscous

    1 Tbls. plus 1 tsp. olive oil
    1 med. zucchini quartered lengthwise, thinly sliced
    1 med. yellow squash, quartered lengthwise, thinly sliced
    2 stalks celery, thinly sliced
    5 mushrooms, sliced
    1 small red pepper, diced
    2 Tbls. fresh parsley, finely chopped
    2 cloves garlic, minced, or 3/4 tsp. garlic powder
    2 Tbls. apple cider or rice vinegar
    Juice of one medium lemon and 1 Tbls. water
    1 tsp. cumin powder
    2 cups cooked couscous, quinoa, brown rice, "Riz Cous," or millet.

Coat a large skillet with 1 tsp. olive oil. Place over medium heat and add vegetables and garlic. Saute until tender crisp. Remove from heat and set aside.

In a bowl, mix 1 Tbls. olive oil, cumin, lemon juice, and 1 Tbls. water. Add to the cooked grain of choice and stir to coat well. Fold in sauteed vegetables and serve warm or chilled.

● **Pancakes**

    1 1/2 cups millet/oat/rice flour
    1 tsp. low sodium baking powder
    2 tsp. cinnamon
    1 tsp. vanilla extract
    2 Tbls. melted unsalted butter
    2 fertile eggs or 2 egg whites and 1 Tbls. water
    1/2 cup amasake

Place all ingredients in a blender and blend. Cook pancakes in a lightly greased or nonstick skillet on each side until brown.

Top with Fruit Compote (p.67) and/or yogurt.

● **Stuffed Kabocha Squash**

    2 med. kabocha squash
    3 cups cooked "Lundberg's" wild rice mix
    1/2 cup chopped onion
    1 cup finely chopped celery
    1/2 cup chopped mushrooms
    4 oz. raisins
    4 oz. chopped walnuts or pecans
    2 Tbls. canola oil
    2 tsp. chick-pea miso
    1/2 cup hot water
    1 Tbls. poultry seasoning

Wash kabocha well and place in 1/2" water in an ovenproof pan. Bake at 350 degrees for 45 to 60 minutes or until tender when pierced with a knife. Remove from oven and set aside until cool enough to handle.

Cut a circular slice in the top of the squash and remove all seeds from inside. Saute onion, celery and mushrooms in oil until tender. Add poultry seasoning, raisins, and walnuts and saute briefly until raisins are tender. Remove from heat and mix well with rice. Combine miso with hot water and mix with rice and veggies. Fill each kabocha with the mixture, packing well. Reheat at 350 degrees for 15 to 20 minutes.

Entrees

● **Chicken Livers in Tomato Sauce**

> 1 lb. organic chicken livers
> 1 onion, finely chopped
> 2-3 cloves garlic, minced
> 2 Tbls. unsalted butter, melted
> 1 small can low sodium whole tomatoes/fresh tomatoes chopped
> 1 small can low sodium tomato paste
> 1/2 cup unsweetened apple juice
> 1/2 cup apple cider vinegar
> 1/2 tsp. oregano
> 1/2 tsp. cayenne pepper
> 1 Tbls. basil
> Pepper to taste

Saute onions and garlic in butter 3-5 minutes. Add chicken livers and saute until done. Combine tomato paste with all liquids, herbs and spices, and pour over livers. Add chopped tomatoes and cook 3 to 5 minutes until sauce thickens. Serve over cooked rice or millet, or a bed of steamed julienned vegetables.

● **Salmon with Dill Sauce**

> 4 salmon steaks
> 1 lemon, plus 1 lemon for garnish
> 2 Tbls. dill
> 3 Tbls. butter, melted
> 2-3 cloves garlic, minced

Combine butter, dill, garlic and juice of one lemon. Broil salmon steaks brushed with mixture and turn over, repeating procedure for other side. Serve topped with remaining dill sauce. Place lemon wedges on the side.

● **Halibut Steak**

> 1 halibut steak, 6 oz.
> 2 Tbls. lemon juice
> 1 Tbls. green onion, sliced
> 1/2 cup shredded carrot
> 1 Tbls. chopped parsley
> 1 tsp. dill weed
> 1 small tomato, chopped

Season fish with lemon juice. Reserve tomato and toss all vegetables and herbs together. Spoon on top of fish. Bake, covered at 350 degrees for 30 minutes.

● Fish en Papillote

    2 firm-flesh fish fillets, such as cod or halibut
    1 scallion, julienned
    1 lemon, thinly sliced
    1/4 tsp. minced fresh ginger
    Freshly ground black pepper

Preheat oven to 350 degrees. Cut four circles of foil about 10" in diameter, depending on the size of the fish. Place each fillet on one of the circles. Distribute the scallion, lemon, ginger and pepper over the fish. Cover each fillet with another piece of foil, and crimp the edges. Bake fish about 10 minutes per inch of thickness. Serve immediately.

● Marinated Seafood Steaks

    Seafood steaks of choice (shark, swordfish, cod, halibut, etc.)
    Marinade (see recipe page 62)

Place seafood steaks in a baking dish with marinade. Marinate 2 or more hours (ideally overnight). Broil or barbecue and serve.

● Salmon with Apples and Limes

    2 salmon steaks, 1 1/4 inches thick
    1 apple, sliced into thin 1/2 moons
    1 lime, sliced into thin 1/2 moons
    1 Tbls. butter
    Freshly ground pepper

Saute lime and apple slices in butter until butter is absorbed by fruit (about 5 minutes). Remove lime ends from skillet and rub over salmon, squeezing juice. Sprinkle on pepper. Broil salmon 7 minutes per side. Serve immediately topped with sauteed fruit.

● Stir Fried Shrimp

    1 1/2 Tbls. sesame oil
    10 large shrimp, cleaned
    1/4 cup green peppers and onion
    1/4 cup snow peas
    1/4 cup red cabbage, chopped

Heat oil in small skillet. Add shrimp and stir-fry for 2 minutes. Add remaining ingredients and cook 3 more minutes.

● Poached Salmon

      5 oz. salmon steak
      1/4 cup chicken broth
      2 Tbls. mirin
      2 Tbls. water
      1 tsp. dijon mustard

Simmer salmon covered in broth and mirin for 8 to 10 minutes. Remove fish, boil broth until reduced slightly. Mix water, mustard and arrowroot and add to broth. Cook until thickened. Serve on a bed of steamed julienned vegetables topped with sauce.

● Fluffy Omelette

      3 eggs, separated
      1/2 tsp. basil
      1 tsp. dijon mustard
      2 Tbls. unsalted butter

Whip egg whites until very stiff in a chilled bowl. Beat egg yolks in a separate bowl with all herbs and spices. Fold yolk mixture carefully into egg whites. Melt butter in a skillet and add egg mixture. Cook over low heat until bottom is lightly browned when edge is lifted with a fork. Place under broiler until lightly browned.

Fill with curried or sauteed vegetables, tomato sauce, Italian chicken livers, etc. Fold and turn onto plate. Top as desired.

● Crunchy Sole

      1 lb. sole
      1 zucchini, thinly sliced
      1/4 cup walnuts, chopped, or crushed rice cakes
      1 Tbls. walnut oil
      1/2 tsp. dried or 1 tsp. fresh tarragon
      Lemon and pepper to taste

Line baking dish with foil, place sole on half. Top with zucchini and walnuts. Sprinkle with walnut oil and oregano. Add lemon and pepper to taste. Bring other half of foil over the top and seal edges. Prick holes in foil with a fork. Bake at 325 for 25 minutes.

• Stuffed Cornish Game Hens

>   2 organic ethically-raised cornish game hens
>   1 Millet Pilaf (see recipe page 35)
>   1 cup unsweetened apple juice

Place game hens stuffed with millet recipe in foil lined baking dish and bake at 350 degrees for 30 to 40 minutes. Baste frequently with apple juice. Bake last 10 minutes at 475 to brown hens.

• Sole Royal

>   1/2 lb. sole fillets
>   3 Tbls. lemon juice
>   1 tsp. apple concentrate
>   1/2 tsp. dill weed
>   1 Tbls. butter
>   1 tsp. chopped parsley

Season fish with 1 Tbls. lemon juice. Heat slowly remaining ingredients except parsley. Saute fish in butter, 1 1/2 minutes per side. Serve fish with sauce and parsley garnish.

• Tuna with Dill Sauce

>   2 cups cauliflower, broken into small pieces
>   4 crookneck yellow squash in uniform chunks
>   1/2 small onion
>   2-3 cloves garlic
>   1 cup no salt chicken stock
>   2 Tbls. mirin
>   1 Large can Tuna

Simmer until tender. Puree in blender until very smooth with:

>   1 Tbls. dijon mustard
>   1 Tbls. dill weed

Place back in saucepan with 1 large can flaked tuna and heat. Serve on a bed of julienned steamed zucchini.

Lemon Chicken

4 organic ethically-raised boneless chicken breasts
1 lemon, thinly sliced
1 Tbls. rosemary
2 tsp. garlic powder

In a foil lined baking dish arrange chicken breasts on top of lemon slices and sprinkle with spice mixture. Bake at 425 degrees for 20 to 25 minutes.

Italian Chicken

6 organic ethically-raised chicken breasts
2 zucchini, sliced
2 fluted squash, sliced
2 tomatoes, chopped
1 onion, chopped
1/2 lb. sliced mushrooms
1 cup unsweetened apple juice
1/2 cup apple cider vinegar
1 tsp. garlic powder
1/2 tsp. cayenne pepper
1/2 tsp. rosemary
1/2 tsp. oregano
1 tsp. arrowroot
1/2 tsp. basil

Place chicken breasts on top of veggie mixture in a foil lined baking dish. Combine all herbs, spices and liquids and pour over chicken. Bake uncovered at 375 degrees for 30 to 40 minutes.

Non-Dairy Zucchini Quiche

1 whole wheat pie shell
1 leek or yellow onion, sliced
2 zucchini diced
2 Tbls. parsley, finely chopped
1 Tbls. olive oil (extra-virgin)
1/2 tsp. oregano
1/4 tsp. black pepper
1/2 tsp. basil
1 Tbls. mirin
3 fertile eggs, beaten + 1 tsp. dijon mustard

Saute vegetables in oil until tender and add mirin/herbs. Transfer veggies to pie shell. Pour egg mixture over veggies and bake at 350 for 45 to 50 minutes or until crust is done.

• Quick Moo-Shu Veggie Wraps

2 to 4 "Tannour" bread <u>or</u> 2 to 4 sheets nori
1/2 cup finely sliced celery
1 cup finely shredded romaine lettuce
1/4 cup peas
1/4 cup finely grated carrots
1 Tbls. sesame oil
1 tsp. mirin
1 Tbls. tamari
1/4 cup water
1/2 cup finely shredded red cabbage
1/2 cup finely shredded white cabbage
1/4 cup finely chopped mushrooms
1 clove garlic, minced, <u>or</u> 1/4 cup sliced scallions
1/4 cup cubed tofu (mirin/tamari marinade optional)

Saute celery, garlic/scallions, peas, carrots, and mushrooms in oil until tender. Add water, then cabbage and romaine until barely tender. Add tofu, mirin and tamari. Serve immediately rolled in "Tannour" bread or nori seaweed sheets.

• Lamb/Veal chops in Balsomic Sauce

4 ethically-raised veal or lean lamb chops
1 cup chicken stock
1 Tbls. olive oil
1/2 Tbls. garlic, minced
1/4 cup balsamic vinegar
1 Tbls. parsley, finely chopped
1 Tbls. fresh mint, finely chopped

In a saucepan, boil stock to reduce volume by half, then set aside.

In a small skillet saute garlic in olive oil until golden brown. Add in reduced chicken stock and vinegar. Reduce volume by half again, over high heat. Add in parsley and mint and set aside.

Broil lamb/veal chops on each side until done to individual taste. Transfer to a heated platter surrounding edges with steamed vegetable of choice and spoon sauce over meat. Serve immediately.

• Chicken Ala King

    2 to 4 organic ethically-raised chicken breasts
    50/50 cauliflower and crook neck yellow squash
    2 cloves garlic
    1 cup chicken stock <u>or</u> 6 cubes frozen stock
    2 Tbls. mirin

Simmer all ingredients in a covered saucepan until tender. Place in a blender with:

    $1/2$ tsp. poultry herb mix
    1 tsp. dill
    1 Tbls. dijon style mustard

Puree until very smooth. Pour back into saucepan and fold in cubed or shredded cooked meat from 2 to 4 chicken breasts. Serve over lightly steamed julienned zucchini. Garnish with paprika.

• Chicken with Artichoke Heart

    4 boneless, skinless, organic, ethically-raised chicken breasts, pounded thinly
    2 cups homemade chicken broth, <u>or</u> 10 cubes frozen chicken broth
    2 cloves garlic, minced
    $1/2$ medium onion, thinly sliced
    2 stalks celery, thinly sliced
    2 Tbls. olive oil
    2 Tbls. mirin
    3 Tbls. parsley, finely chopped
    2 pkgs. frozen artichoke hearts

Saute garlic, onions, and celery in olive oil until translucent. Add chicken breasts and brown on both sides. Add mirin and broth to pan, cover, and simmer 20 to 25 minutes.

Add artichoke hearts and simmer covered 5 to 8 more minutes. Remove cover, add parsley and reduce pan juices to desired consistency over high heat. Serve immediately.

• Potted Chicken

    1 whole organic ethically-raised chicken, cut into parts and skinned (remove all visible fat)
    2 cups chicken stock (See recipe P. 33)
    3 Tbls. mirin
    1/4 tsp. pepper
    1 bay leaf
    2 cloves garlic, minced
    4 carrots, diced
    2 stalks celery, diced
    1/2 onion, chopped coarsely
    2 Tbls. parsley, chopped

Simmer covered 1 1/2 to 2 hours then add:

    2 cups diced zucchini/crook neck yellow squash

Cook covered 8 to 10 minutes.

• Chicken Livers in Brown Sauce

    3/4 lb. organic ethically raised chicken livers
    2 tsp. olive oil
    2 Tbls. mirin
    1 tsp. "Robbie's" worcestershire sauce
    1/2 cup chicken stock

Saute livers in oil until lightly browned. Add remaining ingredients and simmer covered for 10-12 minutes. Add 1 1/2 cups "White Sauce" (see recipe page 66).

    1/2 tsp. garlic powder
    1/2 tsp. "Parsley Patch" seafood blend
    1/4 tsp. pepper

Fold above into the chicken liver mixture and serve over a bed of steamed julienned vegetables.

• Carolyn's Tuna in Cream Sauce

50/50 cauliflower and crook neck yellow squash sliced into uniform pieces
1 can flaked white meat tuna, 8 oz.
1 small yellow onion, skinned
2 cloves garlic, peeled
3 Tbls. fresh cilantro chopped coarsely
1 Tbls. fresh dill chopped coarsely
2 Tbls. mirin
1 Tbls. dijon style mustard

Simmer all ingredients in covered saucepan until tender. Place in blender with /mustard, puree until very smooth. Return to saucepan, add tuna. Serve on bed of steamed julienned carrots/zucchini.

• Tofu Burgers

4 oz. well drained tofu (Chinese style)
1 Tbls. miso (chick-pea is best)
1 Tbls. chopped scallions
1 tsp. mirin
1 tsp. oil

Crumble tofu and add miso and mirin until well mixed. Fold in scallions. Form into a patty and saute in oil preferably in a nonstick skillet. Best served open faced on a rice cake.

• Asparagus with Poached Eggs in Vinegarette

1 lb. asparagus Whisk Vinegarette:
2 to 4 fertile eggs   4 Tbls. lemon juice
                         2 Tbls. walnut/almond oil
                         1/2 tsp. dijon mustard

Poach eggs and serve warm on top of chilled asparagus. Spoon Vinegarette over eggs and asparagus.

• Basil Chicken

4 pounded, organic, ethically-raised, boneless, skinless, chicken breasts, marinated overnight
    in:
1/4 cup finely chopped parsley
1/4 cup finely chopped basil
3 cloves finely minced garlic
1/2 tsp. "Parsley Patch" Italian blend herb mix
3/4 cup chicken stock
3 Tbls. mirin
2 Tbls. "Robbie's" worcestershire

Saute chicken on each side 3-5 minutes in a small amount of marinade until tender. Add remaining marinade and steam covered 10-15 minutes. Serve on a bed of chopped steamed broccoli/escarole.

• Braised Veal Chops with Cabbage

2 ethically raised veal chops (rib best)
2 Tbls. butter
1 cup chicken stock
3 Tbls. mirin
2 Tbls. "Robbie's" worcestershire sauce
2 cloves garlic, minced
2 Tbls. parsley, finely chopped
2 stalks celery, finely chopped
2 cups white cabbage, shredded

Saute veal chops, garlic, and celery in butter until lightly browned on each side. Add stock, mirin, worcestershire, parsley, and celery and simmer covered over low heat 30 minutes. Add cabbage and cook covered 10 more minutes.

• Veal Chops Calabres

2 ethically raised veal Rib/Loin chops
2 Tbls. olive oil
4 cloves garlic, chopped
2 Tbls. lemon juice
1 cup chicken stock
1 green bell pepper, thinly sliced
1 red bell pepper, thinly sliced
1/2 onion, sliced thinly in half moons

Saute veal chops in oil on both sides until lightly browned. Remove to a plate and add garlic, all liquids and veggies. Cook until tender. Reduce liquids over high heat then add the chops to heat thoroughly.

● Meat Loaf

$1/4$ cup parsley, finely chopped

1-2 med. zucchini, finely chopped

2 cloves garlic, finely chopped

2 stalks celery, finely chopped

2 crook neck yellow squash, finely chopped

$1/2$ med. onion

2 Tbls. mirin

1 Tbls. "Robbies" worchestershire sauce

Black pepper to taste

1 lb. ethically raised veal, ground or ground organic chicken

Mix all ingredients well by hand. Form into a loaf shape and bake uncovered at 350 degrees for 45 to 50 minutes.

Soups

• Minestrone Soup

    1 Tbls. safflower oil
    1 small onion
    1 large carrot, sliced
    1 stalk celery, chopped
    1 fresh tomato, chopped
    1 Tbls. tomato paste
    1/4 cup cooked beans
    3 cups chicken broth
    2 cups chopped zucchini/yellow squash/cauliflower/broccoli
    1/4 tsp. celery seed
    1/4 tsp. oregano
    1/4 tsp. basil
    Pepper to taste
    1/2 cup cooked macaroni (whole wheat)

Heat oil in a large stock pot. Saute onion slowly until tender. Add carrots and celery and cook until golden brown. Add tomato and tomato paste. Stir to blend with other ingredients. Add beans and stir slowly. Add chicken broth, herbs and seasoning. Simmer covered for about 20 minutes, or until vegetables are tender. Add cooked macaroni and cook 3 to 5 more minutes. Serve hot.

• Cream of Cauliflower

    1/2 med. cauliflower, sliced
    1 leek, sliced
    2 yellow crook neck squash, sliced
    1 clove garlic
    1/4 tsp. marjoram
    1 tsp. butter or oil
    Water or chicken stock to barely cover vegetables

Place all ingredients in a soup pot and simmer covered for 15 to 20 minutes or until tender. Puree in blender and serve hot.

• Ginger Carrot Bisque

3 carrots, sliced
2 stalks celery, sliced
2 small zucchini, sliced
2 cloves garlic
$1/2$ tsp. grated ginger root
1 cup chicken/vegetable stock

Simmer all ingredients in a covered pot for 20 to 25 minutes. Puree in blender and serve hot or chilled.

• Winter Squash Bisque

2 cups cubed cooked winter squash (acorn, banana, butternut, buttercup, kabocha, Hokkaido)
$1/2$ small onion or 1 leek sliced
Grated ginger to taste
1 cup water/chicken/vegetable stock

Simmer all ingredients in a pot covered for 20 to 25 minutes. Puree in a blender and serve hot.

• Country Pottage

1 potato, cubed
1 carrot, sliced
1 leek, sliced
1 clove garlic
1 tsp. butter or oil
1 bay leaf
Water/chicken stock to cover

Simmer all ingredients in a covered pot for 20 to 25 minutes. Remove bay leaf and puree in blender. Serve hot.

● Curried Carrot Soup with Chives

    1 Tbls. unsalted butter
    1/4 peeled onion, coarsely chopped
    4 carrots, peeled and coarsely chopped
    2 yellow squash, chopped
    1 celery stalk, coarsely chopped
    1/2 clove garlic, minced
    3 Tbls. curry powder
    3 cups chicken stock
    Freshly ground white pepper to taste
    Vegetable seasoning to taste

    Garnish: 2 Tbls. chopped chives

In a large pot, melt butter, add chopped vegetables and garlic, and saute 4 minutes, stirring over medium heat. Add curry powder and cook 3 minutes more, stirring constantly. Do not allow curry to burn. Add chicken stock, turn up heat to high, and bring to a boil. Lower heat and simmer mixture, uncovered, for 30 minutes. Puree mixture in a blender or food processor and serve hot.

●● "Bieler's" Soup

    1 lb. fresh or frozen whole green beans
    2 to 4 stalks celery sliced with strings removed (optional)
    4 to 6 med. sliced zucchini sliced
    1 handful parsley tops (no stems)

Fill a large pot with 1/3 water and add all the ingredients. Cover and cook in rapidly boiling water for 15-18 minutes until the vegetables are fork tender. Then place all ingredients in blender and puree in batches until smooth. Season with any of your favorite herbs, i.e., paprika, oregano, garlic, lemon or basil. Serve hot or cold. **Do not add salt.**

● Quick Minestrone

 1/2 cup pasta sauce
 1 1/2 cups chicken stock
 1 tsp. oregano
 1 tsp. basil
 1/4 tsp. black pepper
 1 pinch red pepper
 1 cup cooked beans (optional)
 2 carrots, sliced
 1 onion, chopped
 2 stalks celery, sliced
 3 to 4 zucchini or yellow squash, sliced
 1 cup cooked leftover rice
 2-3 Tbls. chopped parsley

Place all ingredients in a large soup pot. Simmer over low-medium heat until veggies are just tender. Great to use with leftover rice/beans.

● Meatball Soup

 3/4 pound ground organic ethically raised veal/chicken/or turkey
 Pepper/garlic/basil to taste
 1 1/2 Tbls. "Robbie's" worcestershire sauce

Mix all above ingredients well by hand, and form into walnut size balls. Place in the bottom of a large covered saucepan, add:

 2 cups of shredded white cabbage
 2 cups of julienned crook neck yellow squash.
 1/2 cups of chicken stock or 6 cubes frozen stock
 4 Tbls. mirin
 1/2 tsp. garlic powder (optional)
 1 1/2 Tbls. "Robbie's" worcestershire sauce
 Pepper to taste

Place all ingredients in a large covered saucepan, bring to a boil, then simmer over medium-low heat for 25 to 30 minutes.

• Cream of Celery

2 1/2 cups cauliflower broken into uniform pieces
3 stalks of celery (strings removed) sliced
2 cloves of garlic, peeled (optional)
1 cup or 6 cubes of frozen chicken stock
3 Tbls. mirin

Simmer all ingredients in a large covered saucepan until tender. Place in a blender and puree until very smooth.

• Zucchini Milanese Soup

3 to 4 medium zucchini, sliced
2 cups of cauliflower sliced
2 cloves of garlic, peeled
1 1/2 cups of chicken stock, or 6 cubes of frozen chicken stock
1 Tbls. of "Parsley Patch" Italian herb seasoning
2 Tbls. mirin
Pepper to taste

Simmer all ingredients in a covered saucepan until tender. Place in a blender and puree until very smooth

• Chunky Chicken Soup

Shredded chicken from 4 cooked organic, ethically-raised chicken breasts
1 cup julienned zucchini
1/2 cup of thinly sliced celery
1/2 yellow onion, thinly sliced
1 cup julienned crook neck yellow squash
2 cups chicken stock or 8 cubes frozen stock
3 Tbls. mirin
1/2 tsp. garlic powder
Pepper to taste

Simmer ingredients in large covered saucepan 20 to 25 minutes.

. Mock French Onion Soup

>   2 yellow onions, thinly sliced
>   2 cloves garlic minced
>   2 cups chicken/vegetable stock
>   1 or 2 squares mochi cubed

Place all ingredients except mochi in a pot and simmer for 20 to 25 minutes. Add mochi and cook stirring frequently until mochi "melts." Serve immediately.

● Zucchini Consomme

>   1 tsp. mirin
> $^1/_2$ tsp. thyme
> $^1/_2$ tsp. basil
>   2 cups homemade <u>or</u> low-sodium chicken broth
>   2 cups shredded zucchini

Combine in saucepan, bring to boil, simmer 20 min. Serve hot.

. Quick Basic Chicken Stock

>   4 skinless, organic, ethically-raised chicken breasts
>   4 to 5 cups water
>   3 Tbls. mirin
>   2 cloves garlic, peeled
>   1 small yellow onion, peeled
>   1 handful of parsley
>   2 stalks of celery
>   1 carrot, peeled
>   Pepper to taste
>   1 bay leaf

Place ingredients in large covered stock pot, boil. Lower the heat and simmer for 1$^1/_2$ hours. Remove chicken breasts and save for another recipe (See Chicken a la King p.44, and Chunky Chicken Soup, p.52). Strain liquid to be used fresh or pour into ice cube trays. Freeze and pop out into freezer bags. Store ice cubes in freezer for future use.

• Curried Zucchini Soup

Oil from mister
1 med. onion, chopped
2 med. carrots, chopped
4 celery stalks, chopped
4 to 6 zucchini, sliced
1 tsp. curry powder, or to taste
1 1/2 cups chicken stock
Salt-free seasoning to taste

Mist a medium soup pot with oil. Heat over medium heat. Add onion, carrots, celery, and 1 to 2 Tbls. chicken stock, and saute until onions are soft. Add remaining ingredients. Bring to a boil, cover, reduce heat to low and simmer until vegetables are tender-crisp, about 10 to 15 minutes. Strain vegetables and set broth aside. Place vegetables in food processor or blender. Puree until smooth; add broth until soup reaches desired consistency. Return puree to soup pot. Adjust seasonings. Heat over low heat.

Salads

● **Salad Ideas**

Sliced raw zucchini, cucumber, cabbage, cauliflower, watercress, carrots, jicama, Jerusalem artichokes, sprouts, parsley, and yellow squash are great additions to the normal lettuce salad. Use any of the salad dressing recipes listed or your own favorites (go easy on the oil).

● **Marinated Salad**

>   1 lb. green beans
>   2 cups cauliflower broken into large pieces
>   1 onion, finely chopped
>   3 Tbls. finely chopped parsley
>   1 cucumber, thinly sliced
>   1 cup Seafood/Veggie Marinade (see recipe page 62)

Steam green beans and cauliflower until just tender. Place all ingredients in a bowl and toss. Chill well. Before serving, toss again.

● **Bean Salad**

>   1 cup steamed green beans
>   1/2 cup cooked garbanzo beans or pinto beans
>   1/2 cup sliced leek

● **Dressing**

>   2 Tbls. chick pea miso
>   Juice of 1 lemon
>   1/2 tsp. mustard

Mix dressing well and fold in veggies and beans. Chill well and serve.

● Cabbage Salad

2 cups finely sliced red cabbage
2 cups finely sliced green cabbage
1/2 cup grated carrots
1/2 cup finely chopped apples
1 cup Seafood/Veggie Marinade (see recipe page 62)

Place all ingredients in a bowl, toss, and chill until ready to serve.

● Quick Tabouli Bean Salad

1 pkg. "Cedar Lane" pre-prepared no salt tabouli
1 can garbanzos, rinsed well and drained
2 stalks celery, diced
4 to 6 radishes, diced
1 to 2 tomatoes, cubed
1 cucumber, diced and peeled

Gently fold veggies and beans into tabouli mixture. Serve on a bed of lettuce or in a lettuce lined pita.

Vegetables

● Baked Cinnamon Yams

2 large yams, washed and scrubbed
2 Tbls. unsalted melted butter
1 Tbls. cinnamon
1/2 tsp. ginger powder
1/2 tsp. pepper

Mix all ingredients except yams well. Bake yams in foil at 400 degrees until done (usually 30 to 45 minutes). Remove from foil, slice open and drizzle with butter mixture.

● Chinese Stirfry

1/2 lb. asparagus, sliced diagonally
1/2 cup bamboo shoots
1/2 cup bean sprouts
3 green onions, sliced
1/2 lb. Chinese pea pods
1 zucchini, thinly sliced
3 cloves garlic, finely chopped
6-8 water chestnuts
1 Tbls. sesame oil
1/2 tsp. ginger, grated
1/2 cup unsweetened apple juice
1/2 tsp. curry powder
1/2 cup chicken stock

Place onions, garlic, herbs, and spices in a large skillet and add oil and chicken stock. Saute at high heat for 3 to 5 minutes. Add apple juice and remaining ingredients, cook on high heat stirring occasionally for 5 to 8 minutes or until veggies reach desired crispness..

● Curried Sweet Potatoes

3 to 4 sweet potatoes, cubed
1/2 cup Curry Sauce (see recipe)

Steam sweet potatoes 10 to 15 minutes. Mash and blend with Curry Sauce. Pour into foil lined baking dish and bake at 375 degrees for 15 to 20 minutes.

● Pepper and Zucchini Saute

   $1/2$ onion, thinly sliced
   2 zucchini, thinly sliced
   1 red or green pepper, sliced
   2 to 3 cloves garlic, finely chopped
   $1/2$ tsp. basil
   $1/2$ tsp. pepper
   1 Tbls. olive oil
   2 Tbls. chicken stock
   $1/2$ tsp. rosemary

Saute onion, garlic, herbs, and spices in oil and chicken stock mixture. Add zucchini and pepper and cook covered an additional 5 to 8 minutes.

● Breakfast Zucchini Saute

   1 onion, finely chopped
   3 zucchini, grated
   1 clove garlic, finely chopped
   $1/2$ tsp. basil
   $1/2$ tsp. cayenne pepper
   $1/2$ cup chicken stock
   2 Tbls. unsalted butter
   3 fertile eggs, beaten well

Melt butter in skillet, add onion, garlic. Saute until tender. Add zucchini, basil, cayenne, and chicken stock. Saute until well done. Pour eggs over top and cook without stirring until set.

● Yam Souffle #1

   2 fertile egg whites
   1 large yam, cooked and mashed
   1 Tbls. apple juice concentrate
   $1/2$ tsp. cinnamon

Beat egg whites until very stiff. In a food processor, combine yam, juice, cinnamon, and blend until smooth. Gently fold in egg whites. Pour into a heatproof souffle dish and bake at 375 degrees for 25 to 30 minutes. Serve immediately.

● Yam Souffle #2

 2 fertile egg whites
 1 large yam, cooked and mashed
 1 Tbls. low sodium tamari
 1/2 tsp. ground ginger
 1 Tbls. apple juice

● Spicy Squash

 2 Tbls. vegetable oil
 1 med. onion, chopped
 2 garlic cloves, minced
 1/2 tsp. minced fresh ginger
 1/2 tsp. dry hot red pepper flakes
 1/2 cup chicken stock
 1/4 cup turmeric
 1 Tbls. apple juice concentrate
 1 lb. butternut squash, peeled and cut into 1/2 inch cubes

Place the oil in a large skillet over moderate heat. Cook the onion and garlic until tender. Stir in the ginger, hot pepper, turmeric, apple juice and 1/2 cup chicken stock. Add the squash cubes and cook, stirring for 5 minutes. Cover, reduce the heat to low, and cook for 10 minutes longer, until the squash is soft but still firm.

● Ratatoulle with Rosemary

 1 med. zucchini, sliced
 1 med. summer squash, sliced
 1 med. eggplant, cubed
 3 tomatoes, chopped
 1 red pepper, chopped
 1 clove garlic, finely minced
 1 onion, finely chopped
 2 Tbls. vegetable oil
 1/4 tsp. pepper
 1 Tbls. fresh basil, finely minced
 1 tsp. fresh rosemary, finely chopped
 1 tsp. fresh parsley, finely chopped

In a skillet, heat the oil and saute the onion and garlic until tender. Put the vegetables, herbs, salt and pepper into a casserole dish. Pour the onion over the vegetables and toss well. Cover the casserole and bake in a preheated 350 degrees oven for 45 minutes. Serve hot or cold.

• Eggplant - Zucchini Salad

2 small eggplants, about 1/2 lb each
3 med. red bell peppers
2 med. zucchini diced into 1" pieces
3 Tbls. olive oil
2 Tbls. lemon juice
1/2 tsp. oregano
1 garlic clove, minced
2 Tbls. fresh parsley, chopped

Broil eggplants and peppers for 5 to 7 minutes on each side or until slightly charred. Cool. Remove skin. Dice eggplants into 1" pieces. Seed red peppers and cut into strips. Steam vegetable until tender crisp. In a bowl combine olive oil, lemon juice, oregano, garlic and parsley. Chill vegetables in marinade at least 2 hours.

• Lemon Summer Squash

1 clove garlic, minced
2 Tbls. Fresh parsley, minced
1 tsp. grated lemon peel
2 med. zucchini, julienned
2 med. yellow squash, julienned
1/2 cup chicken broth
1/8 tsp. pepper

Saute yellow squash and zucchini in 3 Tbls. chicken broth until just tender, add remaining broth, simmer covered 5 to 8 minutes. Stir in garlic, lemon peel and parsley and cook uncovered 3 to 5 more minutes. Serve hot, cold or at room temperature.

• Balsamic Zucchini

4 med. zucchini sliced into thin 1/2 moons
1 med shallot, minced
2 Tbls. olive oil
1 Tbls. balsamic vinegar
2 Tbls. fresh mint, finely chopped
Pepper to taste

Saute shallot and zucchini in olive oil until tender crisp (adding water or broth if necessary to prevent sticking). Add vinegar, mint and pepper. Allow to stand for at least 15 minutes in order for flavors to blend and deepen. Serve at room temperature.

Beat egg whites until very stiff. In a food processor, combine yam, juice, ginger and tamari and blend until smooth. Gently fold in egg whites. Pour into a heatproof souffle dish and bake at 375 degrees for 25 to 30 minutes. Serve immediately.

• Blister Potatoes

    2 large potatoes

Preheat oven to 350 degrees. Wash potatoes but do not peel. Slice into 1/4 inch circles. Place directly on a nonstick cookie sheet. Bake for 30 minutes or until potatoes are brown and have a "blister" on top. Remove from oven carefully with a spatula. Brush with Garlic Butter Sauce:

    2 Tbls. butter
    1/2 tsp. garlic powder

In a small saucepan, melt butter with garlic powder.

• Marinated Fresh Vegetables with Fennel

    1 Tbls. oil
    3 Tbls. water
    1 Tbls. apple cider vinegar
    1/2 tsp. oregano
    1/2 tsp. thyme
    1 Tbls. parsley
    6 peppercorns
    1 or 2 peeled garlic cloves (optional)
    1/8 tsp. fennel seeds
    Pinch of celery seeds and salt (optional)
    2 to 3 cups fresh artichoke hearts, carrots, cauliflower, mushrooms, cucumbers, peppers,
    green beans in season.

In a saucepan combine oil, water, and vinegar. Bring to a boil, add herbs, and cook slowly for about 5 minutes. Remove from heat and cool. Steam vegetables until tender. Store marinade and vegetables together in refrigerator overnight. Serve cold.

Sauces/Spreads/Dips/Dressing

● **Vinegarette Dressing**

    1 tsp. dijon-style mustard
    1 tsp. chick pea miso
    1 Tbls. extra-virgin olive oil
    $1/2$ tsp. basil
    $1/8$ tsp. black pepper
    1 clove crushed garlic
    2 Tbls. brown rice vinegar
    1 Tbls. apple juice concentrate
    1 Tbls. water with $1/2$ tsp. mirin

Mix all ingredients well and chill until ready to use.

● **Miso Mushroom Gravy**

    1 Tbls. sesame oil
    1 lb. mushrooms, sliced
    1 onion, thinly sliced
    1 Tbls. arrowroot
    1 Tbls. natural worcestershire sauce (optional)
    $1 1/2$ cups water
    1 Tbls. tamari
    1 Tbls. miso
    Freshly ground pepper, to taste

In a large saucepan, cook mushrooms and onions in the sesame oil over moderately low heat for 10 minutes, until the mushrooms release their juices. Dissolve the arrowroot in the tamari, miso, and worcestershire, stir into mushroom mixture. Add $1 1/2$ cups water, increase the heat to moderate and cook for 15 minutes, stirring occasionally, until thickened. Season as desired.

● Curry Sauce

2 Tbls. curry powder
$^1/_2$ cup water
$^1/_2$ cup unsweetened apple juice
1 onion, quartered
3 garlic cloves
$^1/_2$ tsp. cumin
$^1/_2$ tsp. tumeric
1 tsp. freshly grated ginger

Steam onion and garlic 3 to 5 minutes. Place in a saucepan and add remaining ingredients. Simmer 3 to 5 minutes. Puree mixture in a blender. This sauce is delicious over steamed veggies, over sauteed chicken slices and veggies, scrambled eggs, broiled lamb or chicken.

● Seafood/Veggie Marinade

$^1/_3$ cup apple juice concentrate
$^1/_2$ cup apple cider vinegar
1 glove garlic crushed
1 tsp. basil
$^3/_4$ tsp. dijon-style mustard
$^1/_8$ tsp. ground white pepper

Combine and use as a marinade for any seafood or veggie dish.

● Fresh Quick Herb Dip

2 cups low-fat yogurt
2 Tbls. chopped fresh parsley
1 Tbls. fresh dill weed
1 tsp. chopped fresh chives
1 tsp. fresh marjoram
Garlic (optional)

Blend herbs with yogurt and chill. Serve with raw vegetables.

• Low-Calorie Pseudo Pesto

1 1/2 cups loosely packed fresh basil leaves
1/2 cup loosely flat-leaf (Italian) parsley leaves
2 Tbls. fresh lemon juice with ° cup water
2 Tbls. Olive oil
2 tsp. freshly ground black pepper

In a food processor fitted with the steel blade, process basil and parsley. In a thin stream, as if making a mayonnaise, add the lemon juice and 3/4 cup water. Pepper sparingly. Let sit for at least 1/2 hour before serving. (Keeps 3 to 4 days refrigerated.)

• Special Sour Cream

1 cup water
1/8 tsp. sea salt
4 oz. tofu
1 layer of 12" X 12" cheesecloth
1/2 Tbls. lemon juice

Bring water to a boil. Add salt. Drop in tofu and return water to boil. Remove pan from heat and allow to sit for three minutes. Remove tofu with a slotted spoon and place in center of cheesecloth. Pull four corners of cheesecloth up, twist tight, and squeeze all excess water from tofu. Place tofu, lemon juice, and salt into a blender or food processor and puree until smooth. Yields about 1/2 cup. Use whenever sour cream is called for.

• Quick Catsup

2 small cans low sodium tomato paste
1/2 cup unsweetened apple juice
1/2 cup apple cider vinegar
1/2 tsp. oregano
1 to 2 dashes cayenne pepper

Place all ingredients in a saucepan and simmer 3 to 5 minutes. Chill until ready to use.

● Herb Blend

1 tsp. each:	dried basil
	marjoram
	thyme
	oregano
	parsley
	summer savor
	ground cloves
	mace
	black pepper
1/4 tsp. each:	ground nutmeg
	cayenne pepper

Combine herbs in a jar with a tight-fitting lid. Store in a cool place up to six months. Use as a seasoning for meats and vegetables.

● Sour Cream Potato Topping

1/2 cup yogurt
1/4 cup chopped parsley
Paprika to taste 1 Tbls. lemon juice

Fold yogurt, parsley, and lemon juice together and top a baked potato. Sprinkle with paprika and serve.

● Baked Potato Topping

1/2 bell pepper, diced
1 Tbls. olive oil
3 sliced mushrooms
1/2 small onion, minced
1 clove garlic, minced
1 Tbls. chopped parsley
Herbs of choice to taste (basil, rosemary, tarragon)

Saute onions and garlic until transparent. Add remaining ingredients and cook slowly over low heat until done. Additional water may be added to prevent sticking at any time. Serve over baked potato with steamed greens or a salad.

• Tomato Sauce

10 oz. can low sodium tomatoes, whole
1 small can low sodium tomato paste
1/2 cup unsweetened apple juice
1/2 cup water
1/2 tsp. oregano
1/2 tsp. basil
1/2 tsp. pepper
1/2 cup finely chopped onions
3 cloves garlic, finely chopped
1 cup chicken stock

Place onions, garlic and herbs in a saucepan and cover with chicken stock. Saute until onions are transparent. Add remaining ingredients and simmer over low heat, stirring occasionally for 1 1/2 hours. This sauce can be frozen or chilled until ready to use.

• Dipping/Veggie Sauce

2 Tbls. mild vinegar
1 Tbls. chick pea miso
1 tsp. low/no sodium dijon style mustard
2 Tbls. sesame oil

Blend vinegar, miso, mustard in a blender while slowly adding sesame oil until thickened.

• Salad Dressing

1/2 cup apple cider vinegar
1/2 cup unsweetened apple juice
1/2 tsp. dry mustard
1/2 tsp. paprika
1/2 tsp. finely chopped garlic
1/2 tsp. basil

Place ingredients in a jar, shake well and chill until ready to use.

• No Oil French Dressing

2 cloves garlic
2 med. tomatoes
1 carrot
1 Tbls. grated lemon rind
1/2 tsp. basil
1/2 tsp. paprika
1/2 tsp. pepper
1/2 cup unsweetened apple juice

Steam tomatoes, garlic, and carrot 3 to 5 minutes. Place in a blender with remaining ingredients and puree. Chill until ready to use.

• Cream Dressing

1 medium cucumber, peeled and seeded
1 1/2 cups low-fat yogurt
1 Tbls. chives (fresh or frozen), chopped <u>or</u> 1 Tbls. scallion tops, finely chopped
1/4 tsp. dried mint, <u>or</u> 1 tsp. fresh mint, chopped (optional)
1/4 tsp. freshly ground black pepper

Puree all ingredients in a blender until smooth.

• Lemon Dressing

1 cup lemon juice
2 fertile egg yolks
2 cloves garlic, very finely minced
1/4 tsp. dried dill <u>or</u> 1 Tbls. parsley, chopped
2 tsp. dijon mustard

Puree all ingredients in a blender until smooth.

Fruits and Desserts

● **Fruit Compote**

> 2 to 3 cups of any fresh, frozen unsweetened fruit
> 1/2 cup unsweetened fruit juice of choice (Heinke's fruit cider blends are nice)

Place in a saucepan and simmer until desired consistency is reached. This compote may be served hot or chilled. You may also use this as a sauce for pancakes, waffles, french toast, or to top hot cereal or rice cakes. Flavor with the following fruit/spice combinations:

> Blueberries: apple juice, ginger
> Apples: apple juice, cinnamon, allspice, cloves, cardamon
> Peaches: apple juice, cinnamon, ginger, apple juice and almond extract.
> Apricots: apple juice, ginger, lemon rind, apple juice and almond extract.
> Strawberries: pineapple juice, vanilla extract.
> Raspberries: "Heinke's" raspberry cider and almond extract (or vanilla.
> Pears: pear juice/apple juice, cinnamon/cardamon

● **Apple Parfait**

> 2 apples, finely chopped
> 2 tsp. cinnamon
> 1/2 tsp. ginger
> 16 oz. plain low/nonfat yogurt
> 12 raw almonds, finely chopped

Mix spices with yogurt and 1/2 almond mixture. Divide yogurt into two portions. Fold chopped apple into the first yogurt portion with almonds. Layer with balance of yogurt and sprinkle remaining almonds between each layer. Chill briefly and serve.

● Fruit Yogurt

> 2 cups fruit of choice
> 3 cups plain low/nonfat yogurt

Puree fruit in blender with yogurt and chill. Flavor with the following fruit/spice suggestions:

> Blueberry: ginger
> Apple: cinnamon, allspice, cloves, cardamon
> Peach: cinnamon, ginger
> Apricot: ginger, lemon rind, cloves
> Strawberry: vanilla extract/almond extract
> Raspberry: vanilla extract/almond extract

● Baked Apples/Pears

> 2-4 rome or pippin apples, or pears, cored
> 1/2 cup unsweetened apple juice
> 1/2 tsp. cloves
> 1 1/2 tsp. vanilla extract
> 2 tsp. cinnamon
> 1/2 cup water

Combine liquids and spices and pour over apples. Bake covered at 375 degrees for 25 to 30 minutes. Serve hot or chilled.

● Creamy Apple Custard

> 2 cups peeled apple chunks
> 2 cups apple juice
> 3 Tbls. agar-agar flakes
> 1 tsp. vanilla extract
> 1 Tbls. tahini

Cook apples in juice until well done and then add 3 Tbls. agar-agar flakes. Cook 3 to 5 minutes stirring constantly. Remove from heat and add vanilla and tahini. Blend and refrigerate until set. Re-blend, pour into desert cups and chill thoroughly.

• Poached Pears With Raspberry Sauce

    4 large bosc pears, peeled (leave stems on)
    1 1/2 cups "Heinkes" raspberry cider
    2 cups fresh or frozen unsweetened raspberries

Place pears and juice in a large covered saucepan and simmer 30 to 40 minutes until tender. Remove pears from juice and then reduce to 1/3 cup over high heat. Cool pan liquid and puree with raspberries in a blender.

To serve, place a small pool of raspberry sauce on a dessert place. Set pear upright on place and drizzle more raspberry sauce over the top.

• French Custard

    2 fertile eggs, well beaten
    1 cup R.W. Knudsen coconut nectar
    1/2 Tsp. cinnamon

Blend well and pour into lightly greased baking dish. Set in water filled pan and bake at 350 degrees for 30 minutes or until a toothpick inserted into center comes out dry.

• Dates Stuffed With Almond Fudge

    8 oz. jar almond butter
    4 Tbls. "Hain" apple juice concentrate (syrup)
    2 tsp. no alcohol, no sugar, butterscotch extract or no alcohol, no sugar, vanilla extract

Puree almond butter, apple juice concentrate, and extract until smooth. Stuff dates with almond fudge and chill. These are for special occasions only.

• Fruit Tarts

Crust: 1 cup oat/millet/rice flour (see recipe, page 11)
       2 Tbls. sweet butter, melted
       1/2 tsp. cinnamon
       1 tsp. vanilla
       Water as needed.

Mix well and pat into small tart pans. Prepare the filling:

       1 1/2 cups sliced fruit of choice
       1/2 cup unsweetened apple juice
       1 Tbls. arrowroot powder
       2 tsp. cinnamon
       1/2 tsp. ginger

Heat juice, spices, and arrowroot until thickened and pour over fruit. Mix well and fill tart shells. Bake at 350 degrees for 25 to 30 minutes.

• Fig Crunchies

       2 cups millet/oat/rice flour
       2 tsp. cinnamon
       2 fertile eggs, well beaten
       1 Tsp. low sodium baking powder
       2 Tbls. unsalted butter, melted
       3 dried figs, finely chopped
       Apple juice, unsweetened, as needed

Combine all dry ingredients. Mix in eggs, butter, and juice as needed to make a stiff cookie dough. Fold in figs and shape into walnut size balls and flatten. Place on lightly greased baking sheet and bake at 325 degrees for 15 minutes.

Variation: Used unsweetened applesauce and chopped apple instead of figs.

● Fruit Crisp

3 cups sliced or coarsely chopped seasonal fresh fruit

(apples, pears, peaches, apricots, blueberries, raspberries, etc.)

3 Tbls. arrowroot

$^1/_2$ cup unsweetened fruit juice of choice

Spices of choice i.e. (cinnamon, ginger, cloves, cardamon, etc.)

8 to 10 oz. fruit juice sweetened granola or 2 packs of your favorite natural cookies.

$^1/_2$ cup apple juice concentrate or "Mystic Lakes" mixed fruit concentrate.

Toss fruit with arrowroot and spices of choice to evenly coat. Place in an oven proof deep dish, or a small dutch oven and pour fruit juice of choice over fruit slices.

In a blender grind granola or cookies to a fine consistency. In a bowl combine fruit concentrate and granola or cookies to form a mixture that resembles a crumb cake topping. Put this mixture on top of fruit slices to evenly cover. Bake covered at 350 degrees for 40 minutes. Remove cover and bake an additional 10 minutes. Serve hot or cold.

● Banana Bread

3 very ripe bananas, mashed

2 cups oat/millet/rice flower (see page 11)

1 tsp. low sodium baking powder

2 Tbls. unsalted butter, melted

2 tsp. cinnamon

$^1/_2$ tsp. ginger

2 fertile eggs, or 1 yolk and 2 egg whites, well beaten

10 raw almonds, ground into a powder

$^1/_2$ cup plain or vanilla/pecan amasake

Combine flour with spices and baking powder. Add eggs, butter, and amasake. Mix well. Fold in bananas and nuts, pour into a lightly greased baking pan. Bake at 325 degrees for 30 to 40 minutes or until a toothpick inserted into center comes out dry.

• Sweet Potato Pie

>1 whole wheat pie shell
>3 cups yams, baked well and mashed
>1 Tbls. cinnamon
>1/2 tsp. allspice
>1/8 tsp. cloves
>1/8 tsp. nutmeg
>3 fertile eggs
>1 cup plain amasake

Puree together in a food processor until very smooth. Pour into pie shell and bake 1 hour at 350 degrees. Chill and serve.

• Cream Delight Pudding

>3 cups almond amasake or vanilla/pecan amasake
>3 Tbls. agar-agar flakes
>1/4 cup unsweetened carob chips (optional) or 1/4 cup chopped pecans (optional)

Heat amasake and agar to slow boil, stirring often until agar is dissolved. Refrigerate until set, then blend in blender. Fold in carob chips or pecans (optional) and pour into dessert cups. Chill at least 1 hour. Can be served with a garnish of carob curls using a potato peeler on a bar of unsweetened carob.

• Fruit Gems

>1 cup oat flour
>1/2 cup peach/apricot puree
>1/2 tsp. almond extract
>1/4 cup coconut flakes, unsweetened (optional)
>Apple juice as needed to form dough

Mix together well in a food processor to form a very stiff dough. Form into walnut size balls and chill.

• Peach Moose With Raspberry Sauce

Peach Mousse:

> 4 large ripe peaches, skinned
> 2 1/2 cups "Heinke's" peach cider or peach juice
> 5 to 6 Tbls. agar-agar flakes
> 1 tsp. lemon zest
> 1 tsp. no-sugar vanilla extract

Cook peaches in cider until barely tender. Remove peaches from liquid and place in a blender with just enough pan juice to puree well. Add agar-agar to peach juice, bring to a boil, then reduce to simmer for 20 minutes, stirring constantly. Remove from heat and stir in vanilla, lemon zest, and peach puree. Chill until firm and re-blend in a food processor until smooth. Serve in parfait glasses topped with raspberry puree and fresh mint garnish.

Raspberry Puree:

> 2 cups fresh or frozen unsweetened raspberries
> 1 1/2 cups "Heinke's" raspberry cider or juice.

Reduce raspberry juice to 3/4 cup by boiling. Cool and puree well with raspberries in a blender.

• Oat Bran Muffins

> 1 fertile egg white, stiffly beaten
> 2 Tbls. butter (raw, unsalted), melted
> 1 1/2 cups fruit puree, apple sauce, fruit compote, or favorite similar fruit

Mix together well and fold into:

> 1 1/2 cups oat bran

Pour into muffin cups (lined with muffin papers) and bake at 325 degrees for 12 to 15 minutes.

● *Sample Menus*

Monday:

B: Oatmeal with peach compote

L: Small green salad with vinegarette dressing
       Cold poached salmon with apples and limes

Snack: Fresh fruit

D: Italian chicken
       Rice pilaf
       Cream of cauliflower soup

Tuesday:

B: Fluffy omelette with sauted peppers and zucchini

L: Tabouli bean salad with pitas

S: Rice cakes with fruit conserves

D: Tuna in cream sauce on a bed of steamed,
       Julienned zucchini

Wednesday:

B: Millet with sliced bananas and
       Nonfat yogurt

L: Sliced turkey wrapped around
       Steamed carrot/broccoli/yellow squash spears, spread with mustard

S: Oat bran muffin

D: Cream of celery soup
       Meat loaf
       Steamed swiss chard tossed with herbs of choice

Thursday

B: Pepper or zucchini saute with rye toast

L: Minestrone soup and eggplant/zucchini salad

S: Fresh fruit

D: Lamb/veal chops in balsamic sauce
Steamed julienned carrots and green beans

Friday

B: Five minute grain custard

L: Soba salad

S: Banana bread

D: Meat ball soup
Steamed asparagus with dijonaise sauce

Saturday

B: No flour pancakes with apple compote

L: Quick moo shoo veggie wraps

S: Fresh fruit

D: Millet pilaf
Spicy squash
Variety of steamed greens with butter & herbs
Peach mousse with raspberry sauce

Sunday

B: Van's waffles with fruit compote

L: Nondairy zucchini quiche
Green salad with french dressing

S: Oat bran muffins

website: www.healingessences.com
email: info@kaarenjordan.com
(805) 245-9908